Career Succ...

for Nurse Educators

MW01063002

Career Success Strategies
for Nurse Educators

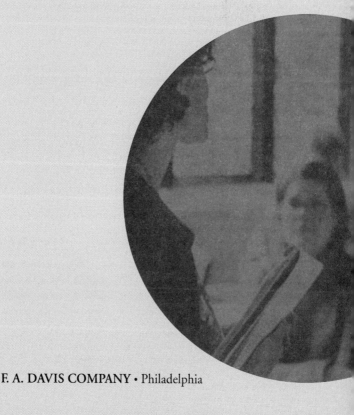

Joyce J. Fitzpatrick, PhD, FAAN, MBA
Professor, Case Western Reserve University
Cleveland, OH

and

Kristen S. Montgomery, PhD, RN
Former Assistant Professor, University of South Carolina
Columbia, South Carolina

F. A. DAVIS COMPANY • Philadelphia

F. A. Davis Company
1915 Arch Street
Philadelphia, PA 19103
www.fadavis.com

Printed in the United States of America

Last digit indicates print number: 10 9 8 7 6 5 4 3 2 1

Acquisitions Editor: Joanne P. DaCunha, RN, MSN
Development Editor: Jennifer Watson

As new scientific information becomes available through basic and clinical research,
recommended treatments and drug therapies undergo changes. The author(s) and publisher have done everything possible to make this book accurate, up to date, and in
accord with accepted standards at the time of publication. The author(s), editors, and
publisher are not responsible for errors or omissions or for consequences from application of the book, and make no warranty, expressed or implied, in regard to the contents
of the book. Any practice described in this book should be applied by the reader in
accordance with professional standards of care used in regard to the unique circumstances that may apply in each situation. The reader is advised always to check product
information (package inserts) for changes and new information regarding dose and
contraindications before administering any drug. Caution is especially urged when
using new or infrequently ordered drugs.

Library of Congress Cataloging-in-Publication Data

Fitzpatrick, Joyce J., 1944–
    Career success strategies for nurse educators/Joyce J. Fitzpatrick, Kristen
Montgomery.
        p. ; cm.
    Includes bibliographical references and index.
    ISBN-13: 978-0-8036-1402-4 (pbk. : alk. paper)
    ISBN-10: 0-8036-1402-4 (pbk. : alk. paper)
    1. Nursing schools—Faculty—Vocational guidance. I. Montgomery, Kristen,
1972– II. Title.
    [DNLM: 1. Faculty, Nursing. 2. Career Choice. 3. Education, Nursing.
4. Vocational Guidance. WY 19 F559c 2006]
    RT90.F58 2006
    610.73071'1—dc22   2006004247

Contents

Part 2
Your Curriculum Vitae (CV)   39

Part 3
Preparing for the Interview: Getting Ready to Get Ready!   49

Part 4
Surviving Your Initial Years as a Faculty Member: Knowledge Is Power!   63

Part 5
Career Success Strategies for Clinical Faculty   77

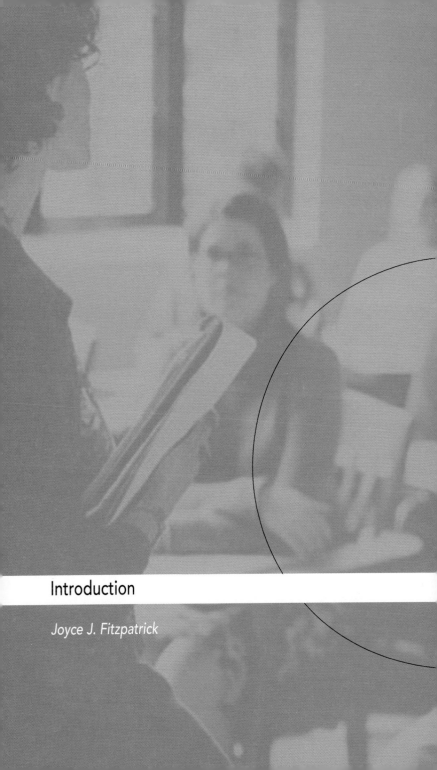

Introduction

Joyce J. Fitzpatrick

Why Should I Read This Book?

This book is designed to help you, the nursing professional, decide if you want to pursue a career in academia. Teaching is a career choice that has a bright future. In 2003–2004, for example, nearly 16,000 prospective nursing students were turned away because of the shortage of nursing faculty (AACN, 2004). This high demand for faculty is expected to increase, as many faculty members in current positions are nearing retirement.

If you are already employed in an academic setting, this book will help you better understand academia and your choices within this system. You are not alone in wishing you had had this information before taking a teaching position. We have found that many current faculty members have not used the strategies included here, mainly because they did not have the background information to make informed choices. Our basic premise is that the more information you have going into a new faculty position or remaining in your current one, the less frustration you will experience. Knowledge is very powerful! It will give you an understanding of how best to navigate the multifaceted academic world of nursing, and it will empower you to choose your career path wisely by using the essential resources at hand.

If you have experienced the academic world only as a student, you may have many questions about academic life and careers. The answers to these questions are generally not relevant to you as a student, but they are important to you in your faculty role. So if you are interested in a new career, one that has a different set of rules than that of the clinical practice environment, there are several dimensions of academic life that will be relevant.

What Is the Academic Life All About?

Nurses are prepared as clinicians; they enter nursing to care for others; often, they gravitate toward the fast-paced, hectic professional lifestyle of clinical practice or the more independent delivery of services in primary care. Most expert clinicians have not been socialized into the academic role, although more and more nurses prepared at the master's degree level are being recruited for clinical faculty positions.

Some of you may have specifically chosen to go into nursing education and prepared yourself for the role by taking a sequence of education courses. You may have earned a PhD and prepared yourself as a nurse researcher, planning to teach and do research at an academic institution. More recently, with the introduction of the Doctor of Nursing Practice (DNP) degree for advanced practice nurses, some of you may have chosen this degree to prepare yourself for clinical teaching. No matter what your previous preparation or your path that led to this career choice, there are undoubtedly some issues that have not yet been discussed with you.

Different Types of Institutions

Academic institutions in which there are nursing programs range from community colleges to research-intensive universities. There are a number of factors that you need to consider in choosing which type of institution fits your career goals: your educational and clinical background and preparation; your short- and long-term goals and how these goals match those of a particular institution; and the personal reasons why a particular institution is appealing to you, e.g., proximity to family and friends.

The three basic types of institutions that you should know about are community colleges, colleges, and universities. Within each type of institution, the nursing program itself can be a program, a department, a school, or a college. So you will need to assess the basic type of academic institution as well as the type of nursing unit within the institution. This information will be important to you at all levels of your academic career. It will tell you the degree of autonomy of the nursing unit and indicate something about the peers you will be working with and the faculty colleagues who will participate in your evaluation. Community colleges generally do not require the doctoral degree for initial appointment to the faculty, although more and more of them are expecting faculty to be pursuing the doctorate if they do not already have one. Colleges and universities require the doctorate for most of their faculty, but this does not mean that you cannot get a faculty position without a doctorate, especially if you are enrolled in a doctoral program. The demand for doctoral preparation is directly related to the shortage of faculty in your clinical specialty area. For example, there is presently a great need for faculty in neonatal nursing at some universities, so expert clinicians with master's degrees in nursing are sought for these teaching positions. Of course, both clinical specialization and a doctorate would make you an even more attractive and competitive candidate.

Community colleges are often the first-level preparation. In nursing, community colleges are primarily sites where associate degree in nursing (ADN) programs are housed. But there are some community colleges that also offer programs to prepare the licensed practical nurse (LPN) and some that offer bridge programs for the registered nurse (RN) who wants to obtain a baccalaureate degree in nursing or in other related fields.

Universities also come in many sizes and are both private and public. Some universities have multiple campuses, as do some community colleges. Many universities have teaching and research as their primary mission. Thus, as a faculty member in a university you would be expected to engage in research and scholarship, and this would be part of the evaluation process.

Public institutions are established by legislation and are ultimately governed by the state, county, or city. Private institutions may receive some support from public sources (e.g., targeted funds for special programs or for research), but most funding is from nongovernment sources. This private funding can come from religious organizations. The religious organization may own the institution, or the institution may be a church-affiliated college or university. Many universities began with religious organization support but then developed independently. Most private colleges and universities are independent; they obtain their support from individuals and from any other private means, e.g., foundations and corporation grants. Many of these academic institutions maintain an endowment in order to fund themselves in perpetuity. In the case of endowment support, only the interest that is generated from investment of the funds is used to support current programs or current operations. Private institutions have various levels of endowments. Of course, those with the largest endowments are often the oldest and may be the most versatile in terms of program support or scholarship support offered to students.

The type of institution will affect its mission and goals. For example, public institutions must serve the constituents of the public body funding them. In the case of nursing, they may need to prepare nurses for the state or local area. While this may not be at the exclusion of other goals, it would be a primary goal. The church-supported institutions will have missions and goals that are consistent with the parent body. Independent private institutions have more flexibility in their missions and goals as the constituents are generally not directly involved in governance. There are always exceptions to these general statements, so you need to examine each specific institution before coming to a conclusion about its type and governance structure.

Before accepting a position at an academic institution, you will want to know its history, type, size, and the sources of financial support. The most complete source of information about types of academic institutions is provided by the Carnegie Foundation for the Advancement of Teaching (www.carnegiefoundation.org). The 2005 classification describes types of institutions within each of the following categories: doctorate-granting institutions (includes intensive and extensive research universities); master's colleges and universities (categories I and II); baccalaureate colleges (liberal arts colleges and general colleges); baccalaureate/associate's colleges; associate's colleges; and specialized institutions. Additional information will be available to you through the institution's annual report and/or on its Web site, often consisting of a brief history and mission and goals of the institution. You will then want to know about the nursing program in relation to these facts about the overall institution. For example, it would be good to know if the nursing program has a larger enrollment than the remainder of the college combined; this is sometimes the case and may place the nursing program in a good position for obtaining support. You may wonder why you need to know all of this before accepting a position. At some point you will discover the relevance in relation to the type of students accepted into the program and/or the effect of the overall mission and goals on the educational program itself.

Is it easy to move from one type of academic environment to another? As with many other questions in planning an academic career in nursing, the only honest answer is that "it depends" on many other factors, not the least of which is the current shortage of nurse faculty in all schools/departments of nursing. It is not always easy to move from the lower-level academic institutions (associate's colleges) to the higher-level institutions (doctoral-granting institutions), but moving in the other direction is often easy, assuming that you have the basic qualifications for a particular position.

The Structure of Colleges and Universities

Colleges and universities have similar structures, although for publicly supported institutions there is the added requirement that there be some accountability to the funding body, e.g., the state, county, or city. The chief executive officer (CEO) of colleges and universities is the president (or chancellor in some of the larger multisite universities), who reports to a board of trustees (in the case of public institutions, this may be the board of education or board of regents for education at the state level or similar bodies at the local levels). The administrative officers include a provost or vice president for academic affairs; several other vice presidents, depending on the size of the institution (e.g., vice presidents of human resources, information technology, research, development, or institutional advancement are common positions in many universities), and the deans of the schools or colleges within the institution.

Depending on the overall size of the academic institution, the nursing program could be a free-standing school or college within the university, or it could be a school within another college. There are nursing programs within liberal arts colleges as well as within schools of education. Sometimes the nursing program is part of a school of health sciences, and within large universities it is part of a health science complex that includes, for example, the schools of medicine, dentistry, and pharmacy. Even if the school of nursing (SON) is part of a university that includes other health science schools, with a vice president of health sciences, it is possible that the dean of nursing reports

6

directly to the provost rather than to the vice president of health science. There are many variations within the structures of universities; some are based on historical precedent, and some are based on operational issues.

It is important for you to know the administrative structure of the college or university and to ascertain the relevance that this structure might have to the nursing unit. If the head of nursing reports directly to the provost or academic vice president, the issues that individual will be concerned about will be those of other nonscience academic units on campus, e.g., psychology or history. If the head of nursing reports to the vice president of health, the issues of concern will most likely be more focused on the health professions. In some ways, nursing bridges both the nonhealth and the health fields as in the other health fields, such as medicine, there are not PhD programs, while there are PhD programs in nursing, thus aligning nursing with the basic science disciplines. Yet the majority of the education of nurses is at the basic and advanced-practice level (and most of that is at the basic level). Thus, many of the clinical academic issues are more similar to those of other health science schools. The head of the nursing unit and the faculty often have to bridge the two areas.

Most colleges and universities are further organized into academic departments. In smaller nursing schools, the entire program may be one academic department, and the head of nursing may serve as the department chair. In larger SONs there may be several departments. These departments are labeled differently depending on the conceptualization that underlies nursing at that school. For example, there are nursing departments that follow the traditional model of organization, i.e., parent-child, community health, etc, and there are departments of acute care nursing, chronic care nursing, etc. There are many differences across institutions.

There are faculty structures within colleges and universities as well as administrative structures. Most often there is a faculty senate that is the governing body for academic issues that are the purview of the faculty to determine. This includes such key issues as the content of academic programs and the criteria for promotion and tenure of faculty. The faculty senate is chaired by a faculty member, and most often each academic unit has elected representatives. Within the faculty senate there are several committees, e.g., personnel committee, budget committee, that have responsibility for some aspect of the faculty functioning. These committees report to the overall faculty senate. There are differences in the level of faculty governance within colleges and universities, and these often change over time.

As you consider a position, you should review the overall governance structure of the college or university and determine if the type of structure will enhance or hinder your own progress and academic development. It will be helpful to know the tenure of the key administrative staff and their academic backgrounds. Also, it is important to review both the process for election to the faculty governing body and to review the bylaws of the overall institution and the faculty bylaws. You also should consider the reporting relationship of the head of the nursing program. Only you can determine if these many factors will affect your own scholarship and teaching.

The Role of the Administrative Head of the Nursing Program

The head of the nursing program has a great deal of responsibility for the academic unit. This individual may have associate and/or assistant deans working as part of the administrative team, or in smaller institutions the head of the nursing unit is the only administrator. If the person holds the title of dean, that person is responsible for the finances for the school as well as for ensuring that the academic programs meet all the criteria for approval (e.g., by the state board of nursing for prelicensure programs) and for accreditation (for both prelicensure and advanced practice and all master's-level graduate programs). The dean must also represent the school as a member of several bodies, at the university, local, state, regional, and national levels.

As the fiscally responsible person for the nursing unit, the head of the program is often charged with finding new sources of financial support for the school, in addition to tuition income. Thus, many heads of nursing units not only participate in writing grants but also do fundraising among potential individual donors, including alumni of the program. At the same time, there is strong encouragement for faculty members to secure outside funding for the projects of their scholarship and research. The pressure to obtain outside support is greatest when enrollments are down, as there is less tuition money. The grants that can be obtained are those from both public and private sources. Public funding can come from federal agencies, such as the National Institutes of Health (for research funding) and the Health Resources Services Administration (for program grants). There are a number of private foundations at the local, regional, and national level that support nursing and health-care projects.

As the administrator of the unit, the nursing head has the responsibility for all human resource issues, including faculty contractual agreements. These agreements for appointment must conform to the bylaws of the faculty and the policies of the university, but often the head of the nursing unit has some flexibility in the terms of the appointment; that is, whether to offer a multi-year or 1-year contract or how to set the initial salary within the overall university guidelines. If the nursing school is large, the head of nursing will rely on the recommendations of the department chairs or the associate or assistant deans.

The nursing head also has responsibility for all contractual relationships between the school or department and other institutions such as hospitals and health-care agencies for student clinical experiences. Again, within larger institutions, this work may be delegated to others: assistant or associate deans, program directors, or department chairs. But when problems occur, it is the nursing head who must get involved to address the issues.

The nursing head also represents the school or program to community constituents. This may involve public speaking and presentations to the media regarding nursing and health-care issues. The nursing head is the spokesperson for nursing for that academic institution and may be called upon for many related and some seemingly unrelated activities. Some larger SONs have their own in-house public relations staff in order to assist the head of nursing in responding to the media and other constituents.

You should be aware of the overall responsibilities of the head of the nursing unit and conserve the time that you request from that person. It is important that you understand the structure of the nursing unit within the school or college so that you clearly go through the appropriate channels before approaching the dean or head of nursing. You will want to be certain that you have exhausted all other avenues of consideration before you bring a specific request to the attention of the dean. It is also important for you to know the overall responsibilities of the head of nursing in case there are any requests that come directly to you. For example, it is possible that you will be approached by a member of the administration of the hospital in which you are doing clinical instruction. You might also be approached directly by members of the media, depending on your area of expertise. You should always inform the members of the administrative staff, including the head of nursing, when such approaches occur. It is your responsibility to make sure that you communicate appropriately with those who have administrative responsibility for the school. If in doubt, you should always ask for advice on how to approach a particular topic. There should be no surprises.

What Are the Roles and Responsibilities of a Faculty Member?

Teaching is an important role, but being a member of a faculty of nursing carries other responsibilities as well. Generally, the faculty role includes teaching, scholarship, and professional service. The expectations for each of these components and the amount of time devoted to each will depend on the nature of the academic institution and the particular position you assume within that institution. Teaching can be at the basic level, i.e., with students who are not yet nurses but who want to become nurses; at the completion level, i.e., preparing those who are already licensed as nurses, either LPNs or RNs, to complete another program; at the graduate level, including basic master's-level classes, advanced practice classes, or doctoral-level classes. The level of your teaching will depend on your academic qualifications, clinical or research experience, and previous teaching experience. You should never accept a teaching assignment for which you do not have the basic qualifications, including the clinical and/or content expertise in that particular area.

Scholarship includes both clinical scholarship, e.g., evaluation of clinical interventions or programmatic initiatives, and research. As a faculty member, you will be expected to formally communicate your scholarship to the community of scholars in nursing. This may take the form of publications or scholarly presentations at the local, regional, national, and international level. The expectations for your scholarship will vary according to the level of the institution. Research-intensive institutions have more rigorous expectations. Because these expectations are not always explicit, you should ask questions about the evaluation criteria that will be used by those measuring your performance. Professional service is the component that is least likely to be explicit in the delineation of faculty responsibilities. Professional service includes all of your activities at the level of professional organizations as well as volunteer experiences at the community level. For example, if you are an officer in your state nurses association or a board member of a local not-for-profit health-care organization, this activity would be included as part of your professional service credentials.

What If I Want to Be in an Academic Environment to Do Research Rather Than Teach?

Most academic institutions require faculty to do some teaching in addition to research. The exception to this would be if you are hired into a research scientist position, which is a position that is sometimes available at the research-intensive SONs. If you are interested in a research position rather than some combination of teaching and research, the most likely places for you are the SONs that have large amounts of National Institutes of Health (NIH) research funding. Each year the National Institute of Nursing Research (NINR) posts on its Web site a list of the top SONs according to the amounts of research funding they have received. Contact these institutions to inquire about opportunities for a research-only position. In addition to research scientist positions they may have support for predoctoral or postdoctoral researchers. Either of these options would allow you to focus your career on research rather than teaching.

Tenure Versus Nontenure Positions

Tenure continues as a much discussed and debated topic in academic circles, with equal proponents for and against the process, for a variety of reasons. While the number of tenured faculty members has declined over the past decade, the process itself is not likely to be abolished. Tenure is the right to due process accorded to faculty members who meet certain criteria established by an academic institution. It is not a lifetime guarantee of employment, although it is commonly misunderstood to guarantee continuous employment. Basically, it means that a college or university cannot fire a tenured professor without presenting evidence that the professor is incompetent or behaves unprofessionally, or that an academic department needs to be closed, or that the school is in serious financial difficulty. Nationally, about 2% of tenured faculty is dismissed in a typical year (www.nea.org, 2005) and less than one-third of faculty is tenured as of 1999 (National Center for Education Statistics, 2000). Although the process of tenure is predominant at research institutions and larger colleges and universities, it also exists at the community college or associate's college level. If you are tenured at one institution, it is easier to move to a tenured position at another institution. However, some institutions will never grant tenure to incoming faculty members, no matter their academic rank and tenure status at their previous institution. So achieving tenure at one institution is not a lifetime guarantee of employment at that institution and does not always guarantee tenure at another institution.

Obtaining tenure almost always requires scholarly productivity, most often in the form of publications in peer-reviewed journals. At some institutions that are focused almost solely on teaching, the criteria for tenure might be focused on the outcomes of teaching alone. In these cases, excellence in teaching may be measured by publications regarding teaching innovations but also could be based solely on one's teaching evaluations.

At the time of your initial appointment, you will be given a choice of whether to pursue a tenure track or nontenure track position. Important factors in determining whether to accept one or the other are one's own career goals and aspirations.

Tenured full professors are at the highest academic rank within the faculty and thus have the most influence. If you are tenured, the university has committed to your continued employment until retirement, unless unusual financial exigencies occur. Faculty at other ranks, i.e., associate professor, assistant professor, instructor, lecturer, and teaching assistant, have less control over curricula and other policies and procedures inherent in the faculty role. However, the entire tenure process is one that is highly respected at some institutions and highly contentious at others. Some universities have abolished the tenure process, and some newer universities have never considered it.

Of course, if tenure is not an option at the university where you are applying, then you do not have to consider it for the present, although it may become an issue if you seek employment at another institution. Tenure often cannot be transferred from one institution to another (unless you are at the most senior rank of professor), although the time spent teaching in rank as assistant professor or associate professor may be transferred to another institution. Thus, if the new institution has a pretenure period of 7 years (which is most typical) and you have taught at other institutions (at the associate or assistant rank), those previous years may count as pretenure. You can request to have the previous experience not counted in the pretenure "clock" and begin again at an assistant professor level. It would be wise to make this request if you had no publications and no research funding in your previous position, as these activities are the most important for tenure. You can always submit your dossier for tenure earlier than the 7 years if you are ready to do so. Because the teaching responsibilities are often heavy in nursing programs, it is likely that you will need the 7 years in order to achieve tenure. In institutions that have the tenure track, if you opt for this track and are not successful in achieving tenure, then you will be given a terminal contract (usually 1 year). Thus, tenure and the tenure requirements are not to be taken lightly in your career planning.

It is also important to know that it is not necessarily easy to move from a nontenure track to a tenure track, in the absence of major research funding. Thus, it will be important to you to clearly identify your career goals and to plan your work accordingly. You also should seek the advice of as many mentors as you can before making the decision about the tenure track versus the nontenure track.

Faculty Rank and Criteria for Promotion

There are several faculty ranks that are used in colleges and universities. The most common titles are instructor, assistant professor, associate professor, and full professor (most often referred to as professor). Some universities appoint lecturers, but most individuals in the lecturer position do not have the same rights and privileges as those appointed to faculty ranks. If the college or university has a tenure system, tenure is usually granted at the time an individual achieves rank of associate professor.

In addition to the usual faculty appointments, some nursing schools employ part-time, adjunct, and clinical faculty. These appointments are usually for a specified period (most often per semester) and for a specified teaching assignment. Those appointed to these positions do not have the rights of full-time faculty at the school nor are the expectations for participation in school governance as great.

The primary responsibility of the majority of nurse faculty is to prepare the next generation of nurses, that is, to teach. The teaching role in nursing may involve didactic in-class instruction, clinical supervision, and/or online education. Although most often there is not a formal job description that accompanies the faculty role, most schools or departments of nursing have a set of expectations for faculty members. This may be identified in your formal offer of appointment, or it may be specified in a separate document. This will include your teaching assignment for the year.

As concerns your teaching, you have the responsibility to provide the latest information to the students. It is therefore important that you remain current in your field of expertise; when appropriate, you should maintain your licensure (e.g., as an RN) and/or certification (e.g., as an advanced practice nurse). You will also be expected to know about the latest developments in teaching nursing. You may want to join a list serve that is focused on current issues in nursing education in order to stay abreast of the issues.

As concerns your scholarship as a faculty member, it can take the form of clinical presentations and publications or research presentations and publications. Faculty members are expected to contribute to the disciplinary dialogue in their area of expertise and to develop new ways of thinking about the issues and the content in nursing. Some colleges and universities are very specific about the level of participation in scholarship that is required of each faculty member each year, and others are more general in the expectations that are communicated.

The third area, professional service, generally does not count as heavily as teaching and scholarship in the criteria for promotion, especially at the major large universities that are focused on research. Professional service can include activities within professional organizations or community volunteer work, through health agencies or other groups. You can serve as a member of the board of the organization or provide services through that organization in a myriad of different roles. Another component of professional service includes service on the committees within the school or the university. There are more than enough committees, and you should choose those that fit your professional goals.

Make sure to carefully review all the official documents outlining faculty responsibilities, such as the faculty handbook, the faculty bylaws, and any other documents that may be specific to the college or the university. It also is a good idea to review some of the documents that have been prepared by the American Association of University Professors (www.aaup.org); these documents are available online.

You should also review the criteria for reappointment and promotion within the institution so that you are clear regarding what is expected of you both during this first year and in future years. You should be very clear on your ongoing teaching and scholarship responsibilities and should make certain that you maintain your side of the contractual relationship. If there is ambiguity in the expectations, then you should seek clarification from the person to whom you report, e.g., your department chair or program director.

One of the most important things you can do when you are beginning your academic career is to keep good records on all that you do, whether in the area of teaching (student and course evaluations), scholarship (dates and places where you presented your work or citations of publications), or professional service (activities in the community or within professional organizations). You should keep copies of all letters and e-mail communications about your contributions as well. Begin your files that will catalogue your professional work for your future benefit.

Another important fact to keep in mind is that you should limit your professional service until your teaching and scholarship are well developed. Many nurse faculty members make the mistake in the beginning of their careers of being too involved in academic governance, when this should be done at a minimal level.

Type of Doctoral Degree in Nursing

If you do not already have a doctorate, you should carefully consider the type of doctoral degree that you pursue. Currently, there are two predominant types of doctoral education in nursing, the PhD and the DNP. The PhD degree prepares you for a career in research and is the degree of choice if you intend to pursue an academic position at a research-intensive SON. The DNP degree is relatively new; it is the practice doctorate that prepares individuals for clinical leadership in practice and clinical education. If you know that you want to remain in clinical practice for some of the time or if you know that you want to pursue teaching at the basic or advanced practice level, then you should pursue the DNP degree.

While a doctoral degree in nursing is not currently a requirement for most faculty positions in nursing programs, it is most often the preferred degree, rather than a doctoral degree in another discipline. At a time when there are doctoral programs in nursing available to you in many different formats (e.g., through long-distance education), there should be no reason to pursue a degree in another field. Not all nurse faculty members agree about the best way to prepare for an academic career, so you may find that you receive different advice depending on whom you ask. It is important that you seek advice from a number of individuals, including your former teachers, current mentors, and the senior faculty at the institution where you are presently teaching. You may also wish to review the "official position" papers of the major nursing organizations to determine the rationale for the different degrees. Specifically, the American Association of Colleges of Nursing (AACN) has prepared "position papers" on the essential content for doctoral programs in nursing (www.aacn.nche.edu).

In addition to pursuing doctoral preparation, you should participate in continuing education in your clinical area and in the area of your teaching expertise if it is not a clinical focus, e.g., nursing informatics or nursing administration. You also should consider whether to obtain certification in education through a new program established by the National League for Nursing (NLN). The first examination for this certification was given in 2005.

Academic-Year Versus Calendar-Year Appointment

Some schools offer both academic-year (9- or 10-month) and calendar-year (12-month) appointments. Sometimes the calendar-year appointment includes a year-round teaching assignment, and at times the summer months are considered time to devote to scholarship. Some institutions offer a base academic-year salary with an option to add the summer salary, if you assume some additional teaching responsibilities. Most often, with an academic-year contract, salary payments are spread over 12 months. This is important to know for your personal budget.

It is important for you to consider all of the options before accepting a contract for either an academic- or calendar-year appointment. Factors to weigh include the assignment itself and how it fits your career goals and your personal resources and time schedule. You may want to leave your summer months open for traveling or for personal development or advancement of your scholarship. All of these are important considerations.

The Need to Balance Skills in Teaching, Scholarship, and Clinical Practice

As stated above, the faculty role comprises teaching, scholarship, and professional service. Your specific responsibilities in teaching may vary from semester to semester, but the expectations for scholarship and professional service will remain the same. The general rule to follow is that, assuming your work is of high quality, the more scholarship the better. Your activities will need to be structured so as to accomplish you goals in each of these three areas.

If you are teaching in the clinical area, with either basic or advanced practice students, you may also be expected to engage in ongoing clinical practice. This can be very demanding in terms of both time and energy. It will be important for you to maintain a careful balance in your work, realizing that the faculty responsibilities of teaching and scholarship are paramount to your future academic career.

The Nature of the Workload and the Work Week

While there are differences within institutions, your primary responsibility during the work week is to the classroom and clinical teaching. In some schools there is a requirement that faculty members have a certain block of time set aside for office hours for student appointments. Some public institutions require faculty to be in their offices during the work week, but especially with the advent of electronic teaching, and the virtual office, these expectations have decreased. Rather, it is more likely that you will be expected to be available to students by means of electronic communication. One of the most attractive components of the faculty role is the flexibility that you have; the expectation is that you will accomplish the work, and you can arrange to do this on a schedule that fits your personal life (aside from classroom and clinical responsibilities, which are very structured). This flexibility is particularly advantageous to advancing your scholarship, but you will need to plan the time for scholarship very systematically. Most experts advise that you should write each day, rather than saving a block of time, e.g., a day or morning each week, for writing.

Some schools have very formalized workload documents that are calculated each semester based on the number of credits in the courses taught, the number of students enrolled, the number of clinical hours, and the number of advisees. Other schools have a more informal method of making faculty assignments for teaching.

The Community Expectations

As a faculty member, you will be expected to represent the institution positively in the community, and there may be times when you are asked to be an official representative from the school or university to some particular community group. You will often have the opportunity to serve as an ambassador for the school, letting the public know of the various programs and projects that are ongoing. Most significantly, you will have many opportunities to recruit potential students in the clinical agencies where you do student supervision or in your personal contacts.

So: Is a Career in Teaching Really for Me?

Do you like to help others learn how to provide better care to patients and their families? Has anyone told you that you would make a good teacher? Do you want to influence future generations of nurses? Do you like to show others how to do things, e.g., do you like to show new staff nurses how to learn the system on your unit?

There are few born teachers, so if you think you would like to assume an academic teaching career, it is best to have the appropriate teaching courses and supervised experiences. Many schools/departments of nursing offer graduate-level courses in nursing education, and if you have not taken a course of study such as this, it would be wise to do so. You may also find teaching courses in schools/departments of education, but these, understandably, are not as targeted to teaching nursing. As with other career decisions, the more preparation, the better able you will be to assume the position.

Academic institutions are different from health-care institutions and corporations. Although the workload of faculty members varies with the nature of the academic institution, some part of the faculty role in any institution is that of knowledge development and transmission. You are being paid to think and to impart your knowledge to others, the students. The products and results of your work are measured differently than in other employment environments. For example, you might be evaluated on the basis of the number of articles you publish or the percentage of your students who pass an examination. As you will discover in pursuing an academic career, often the requirements and expectations for you as a faculty member are not as explicit as in other positions. Therefore, it is very important for you to know how to obtain the necessary information in order to decide if an academic career is for you. Much of our advice in this book focuses on having you evaluate your own career goals, including personal strengths and weaknesses, so that you can make a more informed decision about your new academic career as nurse educator.

Accepting a faculty position places you on an academic career path, one that is both exciting and challenging. A faculty position is not just a job but a career choice and a path that can lead to future growth and professional development. Each decision you make along the way influences your future options. Most importantly, you should know that the academic life is rewarding on many levels, especially in the realization that you influence many new clinicians and future academics.

A number of important questions arise that might influence your decision about whether to pursue an academic career. Throughout this book, we have highlighted some of the strategies to ensure a successful career, whether this is your first or your final career position. Each of the strategies is introduced through the identification of a common mistake that faculty members are known to make, with tips provided on how to avoid and/or overcome the mistake. As with most other things you will encounter in the academic world: knowledge is power! In reading this book, we believe you will be empowered by the discovery that thinking about your long-term academic future is an essential short-term strategy that contributes to career success.

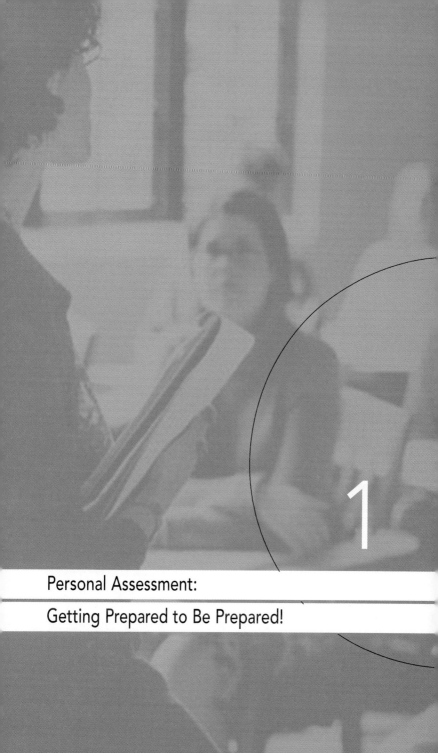

1

Personal Assessment:

Getting Prepared to Be Prepared!

Clarifying What Criteria Are Important in Your New Job Search

Personal considerations often take precedence in our job searches, yet it is important to determine whether they should be given more weight than professional development criteria. The best answer to this dilemma is that both should be considered; you should develop some process for determining the balance or relative weight of each. The most important fact to keep in mind is that you might not want to be changing positions again in the near future; consider that you might want to keep a position for a minimum of 5 years, and make the decision based on what position will serve you best for the long term rather than for the short term. Talk with colleagues who have been through recent job searches, both in academic nursing and other academic fields. If you have the flexibility to move anywhere, consider a session with a search firm, as there are some that have a major investment within nursing, searching for administrators of academic nursing programs, so they can advise you of the criteria used to search for faculty and the relative strengths of the various institutions.

Once you have determined which criteria are important for you, systematically assess the potential places of employment based on these criteria. You can develop your own rating scale to make this assessment. Before you select an institution, compare the relative strengths and weaknesses of all of them. Remember that there is no perfect position, but the goal is to find the best fit for you at this point in your career. Once you have made the decision, make sure you let the other institutions know the choice you made, and never close any doors to future job opportunities.

Tips

- List the personal and professional criteria important in your search process.
- Discuss these criteria with others who have been through recent similar searches and with those who might be knowledgeable about the various schools.

- Assess the strengths and weaknesses of the institutions based on these criteria.
- Discuss these strengths and weaknesses with someone knowledgeable about your field of study, e.g., a mentor or faculty adviser.
- Take some additional time to think about the criteria that you have identified; do not make your decision without taking time to reflect, even if it is only 24 hours.
- Consider your decision in relation to both your short- and long-term academic goals.
- Consider your decision in relation to personal factors, such as proximity to family and friends, attractions of the location, etc.

STRATEGY #2

Defining Your Career Goals

It is common for nurses to begin their careers as clinicians and to move from one clinical position to another as opportunities arise. In fact, the myriad of opportunities within one organization often means that an individual does not have to think about the next step in one's career. It is often the case that individuals are promoted from within, and new positions are created to fit the talents of the individual as well as the goals of the clinical organization.

Once the nurse completes advanced education, either at the master's or the doctoral level and is considering making the shift from a clinical position to an academic one, career planning is essential. This can be accomplished in a variety of ways, both formally and informally. There are businesses and counselors that specialize in career planning, and there are colleagues who can assist. The best place to begin is to ask a local college career planning office for a referral. If you had a mentor during your graduate program, ask that person for advice about career planning. You might also want to ask a colleague who has teaching experience at a comparable institution.

Tips

- Outline (in writing) your career goals for the first year of your faculty role. Start by focusing on one or two activities that you want to accomplish in terms of teaching, scholarship, and professional service as these are the three key categories of activities that are expected of faculty in SONs. (See Appendix J.)
- Do not list more than two activities, as it is important to set realistic goals. It will be better to exceed your goals rather than set yourself up for failure.
- Outline your career goals for the next 5 years, being very specific in the evaluation of what your needs are for growth as a teacher, a researcher, a scholar, and a clinician.
- Discuss both your short- and long-term goals with a trusted faculty colleague or mentor, and listen to their advice about how to modify your goals.
- Identify gaps in your past experiences and what you need to do to fill these gaps.
- Identify what you hope to gain from the faculty experience and how this will support your long-term career goals.

STRATEGY #3

Assessing Personal Connections

It is common for prospective faculty members to underestimate personal strengths and resources or incompletely assess how these resources might be related to a new position. For example, you may be a volunteer at a hospice where students from the school currently have clinical experiences. You may have a neighbor, a colleague, or a friend of your parents who is on the board of the local hospice or the local hospital. You may know those in the community who are in key elected or appointed positions, based on personal contacts or through other community groups. And, of course, you will want to contact anyone you may know who is an alumnus of the college or university where you are considering employment or are presently employed. The more people you know, the more likely there will be some connections to your professional career.

Additional personal resources to keep in mind include special colleagues you know in the national or international nursing community and former classmates or teachers who may be willing to help develop connections for an international exchange program for students or for faculty research. Global connections are extremely desirable at this time in the development of academic nursing at all levels, as nurses have recognized the power of partnerships.

Tips

- Inventory your own personal connections, and analyze how they might be helpful to the SON where you are seeking a position.
- Review the mission and goals of the institution to determine if there are components of your personal resources or personal connections that might be useful to that institution.
- Determine how best to inform the administrators of your resources and personal contacts.
- Determine what resources you are willing to invest to assist the school or college.
- Identify any alumni of the school or university and your connections to them.
- Maintain your connections to others, and expand your circle of influence and contacts.

STRATEGY #4

Developing an Effective Mentor Relationship

Everyone needs a mentor; often, more than one mentor is better. Mentors provide career advice and assist you in your professional development. Many of us have benefited from informal mentoring in our professional careers, but there is an advantage to formalizing the mentoring relationship so that both the mentor and the person being mentored understand what is expected. Your academic adviser in your graduate program may be willing to continue to serve as a mentor for your overall career development. In addition, you may find that it is useful to extend your relationships and find mentors who can specifically advise you in your area of scholarship or in your area of clinical practice. And it is wise to find a mentor in your new place of employment, someone who can help you "learn the ropes" and develop a more thorough understanding of the institution. It is important to be explicit in your request for mentoring if you expect the person to provide targeted assistance. You may wish to have an introductory meeting with the individual to ascertain whether your communication styles and overall values and goals are consistent. Once you have decided that you want the person to be a formal mentor, ask the person and provide information on your career goals and your specific needs for the short term (first year).

Tips

- Once you have identified your strengths and weaknesses, identify the areas for which you need the most mentoring.
- Identify potential mentors from among the leaders in your area of professional need and/or scholarship.
- Identify a career mentor who may serve as an adviser in more than one area of your professional development. (See Appendix M.)
- Identify a mentor in your place of employment, someone who can help you learn the system.
- Be specific in your request for mentoring, i.e., let the potential mentor know your goals and how the mentor can help you achieve these goals.
- If the person you have identified decides he or she is not the best one to mentor you, do not take it personally, but ask for advice about other potential mentors.
- Plan regular meetings with your mentor, perhaps monthly to begin the relationship.
- Once the mentoring relationship has been established, you will have created a pattern of communication that can be continued by electronic means rather than requiring a face-to-face meeting, although some individuals prefer meetings.
- Be cautious, but honest, in your communication. Remember, there is no such thing as "casual" communication in the workplace or in the professional world.

Extending Your Search Broadly and Doing a Comparative Analysis of the SONs

Once you decide to search for a faculty position, it is important to examine as many positions as possible. You can easily do a systematic search for positions among all of the SONs that match your criteria. For example, if you have geographic limitations and are confined to a specific location, search all schools within the boundaries that you have identified, even if they have not advertised open positions. It is important to note that there is often a lag time from the identification of the position vacancy to the time it is advertised, so if you inquire broadly, you may be alerted to some positions that will soon be advertised. Also, even if there is not a current vacancy, there may be an unexpected one that occurs shortly after your inquiry. There is no harm in having your resume on file for future positions.

In undertaking this comparative analysis of the schools you are considering, you will learn a great deal about each of them. It is important that the analysis be organized in some format so that it is easy to capture the data. You may wish to organize the quantitative data first and then proceed to organizing some of the qualitative data. For example, first list the number of students enrolled in the school across all programs, and then list the number in each of the programs. Then list the number of faculty members in the school. This will give you some information about the potential workload, based solely on the numbers. The total number of courses offered adds to the equation as well as the presence (or absence) of clinical and/or adjunct faculty. The number of clinical agencies in which students have experiences will add to your knowledge base. It might even be useful to plot the clinical facilities on a map so that you have an idea of the breadth and scope of the overall faculty workload as related to geographic distances. It is not unusual for SONs to have partnerships that extend to the entire state or that reach beyond the state in which the university or college is located. New partnerships between institutions are common and ever-expanding, and it is important to know about these before accepting a position.

Another dimension of your analysis should be focused on the scholarly productivity of the faculty members and the graduate students within each school. Many of the faculty accomplishments are listed on the school's Web site and should not be difficult to obtain. Not only will you learn about the individual faculty members but you will also learn about the respective positions of the different schools within the national, and in some cases international, academic world of nursing.

- Do not limit yourself to one type of school or program.
- Complete a systematic assessment of the strengths and weaknesses of the different schools; create a grid for capturing both quantitative and qualitative data.
- Note which strengths of the schools compliment the goals you have established for your own career.
- Identify faculty members who could serve as role models and career mentors for you.
- Identify potential faculty colleagues who could collaborate with you on future teaching and/or research projects.

STRATEGY #6

Knowing the Strengths of the SONs You Are Considering

No two SONs are the same, even though they may have similar academic programs, e.g., undergraduate, master's, and doctoral programs. In your search for a position, it is important that you gather as much information as possible about a school so that you can make an informed decision. Although you may not know exactly how the various factors will influence your particular position, you should be assured that they will do so, whether immediately or in the long term. If you are being hired primarily to teach in the undergraduate program, but you have career aspirations to teach graduate students, you may want to choose a school that has both programs. The opportunities to change teaching assignments often fall first to those who are already part of the institution.

In addition, schools are at different stages of their development as organizations. For example, a university may have recently undergone reorganization and the SON could have become the college of nursing and health within the past 2–3 years. This is a major change that permeates the structure and activities of the nursing academic institution. If the school has recently absorbed another institution, e.g., a hospital-based diploma program, this change should also be reflected in the descriptive literature on the school.

Tips

- Review the strategic plan of the SON, including the explicit mission, values vision, and goals. If there is no strategic plan, it is a clue that the organization may not be as systematic in its assessment and development as is desirable.
- Determine if the school's values and vision for the future are consistent with your own, or at least encompass goals you can live with as a faculty member.
- Review the school's Web site, noting how easy it is to navigate and how much information is readily available. Generally, the better schools have invested in dynamic Web site design, and the site should be very easy to navigate. You should be able to find out the qualifications and areas of expertise of key faculty and to get a sense of the strengths and national standing of the school.
- Identify the key faculty within the school, and note those whose credentials are most closely related to your own. These individuals may be your best resources within the new system, and it will be very important for you to become colleagues with them so that you can all learn from each other.
- Identify prospective mentors among the faculty members. Even though you may have a career mentor who is outside this particular school, it is always good to have an "internal" mentor to guide you within a new organization.

Understanding the Reputation of the School

Reputations come and go, yet some components linger on, influencing the present and the future. It is important to know the history and reputation of the school and to ascertain how this influences the specific job and the overall future of the school.

Because reputations are not based on current information, there may be some need to update the community perspective on the school. Individual faculty members may be able to influence or clarify any misunderstandings that exist in the community regarding the history and/or current status of the school. The relationship of the school to the community is important to assess as you will have students placed in health care and community agencies, and you will want to know the overall view of the school and the quality of education.

It is especially important for you to assess the impact the past or future reputation of the school will have on your academic career. It may not matter. If your primary reason for accepting this first position is to gain skills in teaching, as long as the school does not have a marred reputation, the reputation may not be relevant to you. You should, however, keep in mind that this school will always be listed on your curriculum vitae, so you want to have at least some understanding of the school's history and reputation.

Tips

- Ask current faculty members and students about the history and reputation of the school.
- Obtain current and previous school rankings based on the national ranking systems. (See Appendix E.)
- Ask community leaders about their impressions of the school to ascertain their knowledge of history, reputation, and current programs.

31

- Ask key nursing leaders in the state and nationally about the reputation of the school. You can easily track down leaders in nursing through Web sites of professional organizations and SONs. Most nurse leaders will respond to an e-mail query from other nurses. Do not be shy about asking.
- Determine if the reputation will influence your decision about the position.

STRATEGY #8

Knowing About the Students You Will Teach

Do not assume that all nursing students are alike, although they may be more alike than they are similar to other under-graduate or graduate students. Teaching skills that might be useful with second-degree students will not be the same as those needed for 18-year-old freshman students or registered nurses returning for baccalaureate degrees or students who take all their courses online. And, of course, graduate students have different learning styles and different needs, especially if they have been away from the academic environment for years. For example, some graduate students have underdeveloped computer skills and would be best advised to take a continuing education course so that they begin at the same level as others.

Also, you will develop your teaching materials differently if you have 50 instead of 10 students in a class. Before designing course outlines, it will be helpful to know as much about the students as possible. Usually it is possible to find out the enrollment prior to beginning the course. Then on the first day of class, if you do not have any other information, it is helpful to have the students complete a background data form so that you have some idea of their previous experience. On this form you can ask the students to include their career goals and the goals for their learning in this course so that you have an idea of their own assessment.

- Determine how many students are enrolled (on average) in the classes you will be teaching.
- Determine any plans for immediate increases in enrollment in the program, and overall in the school, so that you will know if your class sizes will be increasing.
- Learn about the qualifications used to determine admission and progression of students in the various programs of the school so that you have some general background about the quality of student in your classes.
- Review National Council Licensure Examination scores for the school for the past 5–10 years; this information can generally be obtained from the nursing program administrator.
- Review other characteristics of the student body, especially among students in the program/courses you will be teaching. Much of this information should be available in the state board or accreditation reports of the school.
- Determine what percentage of the students are adult learners so that you can determine if you have the appropriate knowledge to teach these students.

STRATEGY #9

Understanding the Culture of Academe

Many nurse educators have not had an introduction to the culture of the academic world other than through their own student experiences. Often, that view has been limited to the SON, which may or may not reflect the larger system culture. Without a more comprehensive understanding of the university system, including its history in the United States and its structure and processes, faculty members are often unclear about how to pursue various components of their work. For example, a thorough understanding of the processing of grades, the expectations of student attendance, and the student and faculty grievance procedures are all necessary components. It is also important to understand the degree of faculty governance at the particular institution and how this affects the teaching role you will assume. Much of the information that is needed is available in written documents, such as faculty bylaws in which all faculty have access to through formal faculty procedures.

Another important source of information for faculty is the American Association of University Professors (AAUP) available at www.aaup.org. The organization has a long history, since its founding in 1916, of ensuring meaningful faculty participation in institutional governance, including through unionization. The AAUP has position statements on several key issues in higher education, including academic freedom, faculty collective bargaining, faculty workload, tenure, intellectual property, and several other topics. Its Web site will serve as an ongoing resource to you, whether or not your institution has an active AAUP organizational chapter.

Tips

- Review the faculty bylaws for both the university and the SON.
- Review all policies and procedures.
- Review the student handbook.
- Review the faculty handbook.
- Read a book about the history of higher education in the United States.
- Review the AAUP Web site and consider how the position statements influence your academic work.
- Identify how key issues are discussed within your institution, e.g., through the faculty governance process.
- Identify the AAUP presence on your campus, and determine how you want to become involved in order to advance your career and understanding of key academic issues.

STRATEGY #10

Understanding the Relationship of the SON to the College and/or University

As nurses, our perspective has often been very narrowly focused on what is within our immediate control or sphere of influence.

34

We may be so immersed in the "trees" that we fail to see the "forest" or even the environmental resources that nurture the trees in their growth. Further, we are used to nursing and health-care systems and understand more about how these function.

Understanding the structure of the university or college is equally important to understanding the structure of the specific nursing unit within the university. Is the nursing school the only professional school within a college of arts and sciences? Are there other health science profession schools, e.g., medicine, dentistry, public health? How large are these other schools? How do they relate organizationally to the SON? The more you understand about your new academic setting, the better able you will be to understand and interpret any new policies that are implemented and how they affect you and your students. For example, if the SON is part of a health science complex, the university itself may insure the students instead of requiring them to obtain separate malpractice insurance. As a faculty member, you will definitely want to find out about professional liability and insurance coverage for you and your students, especially if you are teaching clinical courses.

Tips

- Obtain a copy of the organizational chart of the university and the SON.
- Ask nurse faculty members at the institution if they know the formal structure of the university.
- Consider the consistency of the official organizational chart and the understanding of those whom you ask about it.
- Inquire about any current vacancies at the level of the university administration and the relevance of these changes to the SON.
- Inquire about the most recent changes in the university administration.
- Review recent accreditation reports of the school and the university.
- Review the insurance coverage that you have as part of the academic institution and your own professional liability coverage.

Understanding the Legal Aspects of a Teaching Position

Several dimensions of the faculty role require knowledge of the legal aspects, from student admission criteria to requirements for graduation. It is important to understand the legal aspects of one's responsibilities as a faculty member. Some SONs have nurse attorneys on the staff, and others rely on the legal department of the university for advice with legal issues. As a faculty member, you will be expected to understand the legal aspects of your role and the responsibilities that you have to the institution and the students. Be certain that you know who the key decision-makers are within your institution and how supportive they are of faculty.

Clinical instruction brings with it an additional set of legal considerations. You should also thoroughly review these before beginning your teaching. Issues such as coverage for malpractice insurance, the rights and responsibilities of faculty and students within clinical agencies, and charting expectations of the staff in clinical agencies are just a few of the topics that should be understood. Prior to any clinical instruction, you should review the contract between the SON and the clinical agency (see Appendix R for a sample contract with a clinical agency). If the expectations and legal responsibilities of your school and the clinical agency are not clearly identified, ask for clarification. You need to be well informed about your legal responsibilities before you need to seek help for a difficult situation.

Tips

- Inquire about the legal counsel for the SON.
- Review the appropriate formal documents, including bylaws, policies for faculty and students, agreements with clinical agencies where students have placements, and insurance coverage (particularly professional liability insurance).

- Discuss any issues you do not understand with the administrators at both the school and the clinical agency.
- Ascertain the process for record-keeping within your school for any issues that might have legal ramifications.
- Understand your responsibility for documentation regarding student process, and be certain you can substantiate your documentation.

2

Your Curriculum Vitae (CV)

Creating the Perfect Curriculum Vitae

The temptation is often to include too much or too little on the curriculum vitae (CV). Focus on including just enough to orient the reader to the highlights and relevant points of your background and career. Although you may include the most information about your present position, it is important that you describe all of your previous positions, however briefly. Whereas it is debatable whether the CV should be tailored to each position for which you are applying, it is important to have a CV that is up-to-date, which can be used to apply for any academic position. It is also important to explain any gaps in professional activity, whether they are due to personal responsibilities, caring for children or a dying parent, or just a time when you escaped to Colorado for a year of skiing. How these gaps in employment are explained is more important than why they occurred. For example, if you took time out to care for children or parents, explain if you had sole responsibility or shared responsibility and what other things you accomplished during this time. Even with gaps in official employment, most people still have some professional activity.

Just as the content of the CV is important, the format and presentation are equally important. (See Appendix K.) Misspelled words are never acceptable; they alert the reader to sloppiness on your part. Other evidence of lack of attention includes an out-of-date list of publications and inconsistent formatting of the citations or references. If you list a person who will provide a reference with his or her formal title and credentials, be certain to list the same for all your references.

Tips

- Do not include personal information on your CV, e.g., marital status, number of children, hobbies, etc.
- Include academic degrees, with the institution and the date of graduation.
- Include formal educational experiences, even if no degree was conferred; describe the course work.

- Include relevant teaching experiences, even if they involved patient education, not student education.
- Do not include RN or other professional license numbers, but do include the states of licensure and/or registration and national certifications.
- Do not include your social security number.
- Include your academic employment experiences, with a brief description of your responsibilities in each position.
- Include your clinical and other professional experiences, with a brief description of your responsibilities in each position.
- Include continuing education that you have taken in the past 5 years.
- Include publications, using consistent format for citation, indicating those that are in peer-reviewed journals.
- Include a list of grants that you have obtained or helped obtain, using a consistent format for each, including the amount of funding and the time period of the grant.
- Include scholarly presentations, using consistent format for each.
- Include a list of three to five names, addresses, and e-mail addresses of persons who are your professional references.

STRATEGY #2

Creating Your Teaching Portfolio

One of the key components for qualification for a teaching position is previous teaching experience. Any evidence that supports your teaching background should be included. Such experiences are: formal courses taught, clinical supervision of students at any level, courses taught as part of your graduate preparation (e.g., a guided teaching practicum), clinical conferences led, continuing education programs conducted, patient and family education experiences, and, of course, any formal evaluations of these teaching experiences. Indicate dates and the number of students involved. It is significant whether you taught 5 or 50 students. Modalities of instruction and the level of the students should also be included. You need not include course or program outlines unless specifically requested to do so. Your teaching portfolio should not be presented with your initial application or inquiry letter; rather, you should indicate that you have a teaching portfolio that can be requested. This portfolio may be what distinguishes you from other candidates applying for the same position. (See Appendix N.)

- Include all relevant teaching experiences in your teaching portfolio, e.g., formal courses taught, continuing education sessions, clinical supervision of students and clinical conferences conducted, and patient and family education.
- Include numbers and levels of students and the time frame as well as the specific teaching methodologies that were used.
- Maintain a file of course outlines of all courses taught.
- Maintain a file of all student evaluations of your teaching experiences.
- Present a summary of your teaching contributions and experiences as part of the teaching portfolio, with an indication that additional information is available on request.

STRATEGY #3

Selecting the Right Persons for References

The general rule of thumb is that it is best to have the most senior and most well-known persons in your discipline write your letters of reference. This, of course, assumes that this person knows your work well and will provide a positive recommendation. Before submitting the names of persons to serve as references, it is important that you speak with them and ascertain their willingness to be references. Also, before applying for any position, alert them to the potential inquiry, and send them a copy of the position description and an updated CV. Their letter can then directly address the components of your background and experience most relevant to the position. It is always better to know ahead of time about a request for a reference. The referee may not be able to meet the time frame for the request. It is better to know this so that you can provide additional names. Consequently, it is better to list more than the minimum number of referees requested. If one person cannot meet the deadline to submit a reference, other persons will be readily available.

Never use friends or casual acquaintances as references. They are likely to write less appropriate letters. The overall goal is to obtain the best reference letters from the most highly placed and qualified academic persons in your discipline or related discipline. In some cases, it is important to match the referees with the nature of the position. For example, if you are applying for a teaching position that involves interdisciplinary work, it is important to have someone from another discipline identified as a referee so that they can speak to your work in collaboration. If you have no contact with your previous faculty or any current faculty, it is time to renew acquaintances. Prepare a letter to your former professors, and let them know of your career history and future plans.

Tips

- Identify the most senior persons with whom you have worked or studied; ask these individuals if they would be willing to provide letters of reference for you.
- Submit names of references at the time of first application for the position.
- Alert the persons who have agreed to serve as referees about the position requirements, deadlines, etc.
- Make sure you keep your referees up to date on your career progress by giving them an updated CV before you request a new letter of reference.
- Inform your referees of the desired format for letters of reference. (See Appendix G.)
- Be certain to thank those who provide letters of reference.
- Keep your referees informed of your decision-making about positions.

Using the Best E-mail Etiquette

Unfortunately, communication in today's world has become very informal, especially with the advent of e-mail for formal communication. All communication about potential positions should be treated formally. There are some administrators who keep all their e-mail and some who print all of them. You will be judged by your communication.

Special cautions are relevant to e-mail communication. Many people do not spell-check their e-mail before sending it. It is always wise to do so. Another issue in e-mail communication has to do with salutations. It is important to be formal in communication with potential employers rather than to assume that a first-name basis is acceptable. Also, use the credentials (degrees, titles) for the persons you are contacting by e-mail.

Before applying for a position online, check the instructions in the position announcement. In some cases, applying online is acceptable, but this is not always the case. If in doubt, inquire before acting.

Tips

• Inquire about the desired form of communication in the application process.
• Treat all communication formally, assuming that it will become part of an official file.
• Always remember that you will be judged on your communication; use all the tools available to you to prepare the most polished letters.
• Make certain you know the most desired form of follow-up for all your correspondence; do not assume that e-mail communication alone is acceptable.
• If the submission of letters of interest and CVs are acceptable electronically, make certain that the formats of your submissions are clear and accurate.
• Inquire about the desirability and acceptance of electronic versions of letters of recommendation before submitting them.

Timing Your Job Search

Whereas most academic institutions have a set time frame for their search for positions for the coming academic year (usually between March and June for the fall semester), many schools of nursing are known to deviate from this general pattern. Many positions are advertised in the early spring semester for positions that begin in the following fall semester of the academic year. This is especially true for tenure positions.

Overall, there is wide diversity in the timing of searches for faculty positions in schools of nursing. Certainly, the current shortage of faculty means that any time might be the right time to search for a faculty position. Most SONs report faculty vacancies; it is often a matter of finding the person with the appropriate credentials to match the teaching needs.

It is best to assume that any time is a good time to inquire about potential positions. If positions are not currently available at a school in which you are interested, you can request that your resume be kept on file for future consideration. This is especially important to do if you know your ultimate career goal is to obtain a position at that particular school. In this case, you might also want to keep an open line of communication with someone who is currently on the faculty at that institution, as such persons often know of openings before they occur.

Tips

- Determine deadlines for any positions that are formally announced, and be sure to conform to any deadlines that have been announced.
- Remember: "Lateness is not greatness".
- Determine deadlines that might be more flexible or dependent on increased enrollment.
- Maintain an up-to-date CV so that you are prepared to respond to deadlines that have a short turnaround.

- Keep a file of past advertisements from the institutions that you are interested in so that you have a sense of the requirements of job applicants and of the general time frame from advertisement to selection.
- Maintain a line of communication with key contacts at the desired institutions so that you learn of any new positions before they are officially announced.

3

Preparing for the Interview:

Getting Ready to Get Ready!

STRATEGY #1

Getting the Position Descriptions or Criteria on Which You Will Be Evaluated

Individuals who are new at faculty interviewing may be hesitant to ask for formal descriptions of the positions or the criteria on which faculty are evaluated. Note that most schools of nursing have at least some of these documents in writing. Thus, it should be fairly easy to obtain them on request. If it is difficult to get this information, that in itself is a clue that perhaps there is a need for more of an infrastructure within the organization.

It is equally important to ascertain if there are informal criteria on which faculty members are judged, beyond the formal job description and the published criteria for evaluation and advancement within the system. Often the best persons to ask about this are the current faculty members, especially those who have been at the institution for some time and those who are in positions lateral to the one you are seeking.

It is easier to meet the criteria for evaluation if you know what they are; the time of your first annual evaluation may not be the best time to find out.

- Request copies of formal documents that are used for faculty evaluations at your level.
- Request copies of formal documents that are used for faculty, administrators, and staff at other levels within the SON.
- Ask questions about informal methods of evaluation or additional criteria beyond the published ones.
- Ask about the process for student evaluations of faculty, including whether these evaluations are posted on the Web, whether they are used in your review for promotion, and how they are considered in annual salary increases.
- Ascertain who will participate in your formal evaluations, how decisions will be made, and who will have the final decision on salary increases and promotions.

• Determine if you will be expected to complete a self-evaluation of your accomplishments and how this self-evaluation will be used in the overall process.

Understanding How the Nontenure Track Fits Into the Overall Structure of the School and University

Many faculty members do not understand the overall fit between the tenure track and the nontenure track roles within the SON. Although some of the specific information should be available in the faculty bylaws, there is undoubtedly some informal information that will also be useful. The guiding principle should be that the more information you have, the better your understanding will be. It might also be helpful to discuss the history of the nontenure track with senior members of the SON faculty.

Different titles are used for nontenured faculty members. There are also differences between schools regarding the expectations of nontenure faculty. Most often, however, the requirements for scholarship are still paramount, but the manner in which this scholarship can be expressed varies. For example, some schools consider the scholarship of teaching or excellence in clinical practice important for nontenured faculty. One of the key differences between tenured and nontenured faculty members is the research expectation; the latter are not expected to secure research funding or necessarily participate in research.

• Review the formal criteria for promotion for faculty in the SON.
• Differentiate the roles of the tenure track and nontenure track faculty.
• If you are considering either a tenured or nontenured position, evaluate the differences in the roles in terms of your career goals.
• Consider the benefits, financial and otherwise, of both tracks.

- Discuss your career goals and your faculty role options with mentors and senior faculty members.
- Inquire about nontenured positions within other schools on campus to determine if the faculty expectations are similar.

STRATEGY #3

Understanding the Support of Key Players, Including University Administrators and Community Leaders

Just as many nurses are very knowledgeable about the organizational structures of health-care systems, they also may be aware of the formal and informal support for nursing within those structures. Such awareness is equally important to ascertain within the academic environment. Where are the champions of nursing, or are there any? If there are not current champions, is there interest among the academic nursing leaders in developing relationships with the key administrative leaders in the university and within the larger community?

What support is there for nursing generally (not just for this SON) within the larger community? Are there key nurses on boards of directors of community agencies related to health and wellness? Do community leaders understand nursing within the context of medicine or as a separate, distinct discipline? The community perception of the SON will help you understand how various constituents react both to you as a faculty member and to your students.

You also will want to determine if the nursing school or department is identified within the overall publicity and public relations initiatives of the institution or whether the nursing unit has to struggle constantly for recognition. Ask the dean or director about this, and review formal public relations documents to determine the attention given to the nursing unit.

- Inquire about the support for nursing among key academic leaders and community leaders.

- Review the lists of boards of directors for key health-care organizations in the community to determine if there are nurse members.
- Review the lists of boards of directors for the clinical agencies where students work to determine if there are any nurse members.
- Evaluate the participation of the faculty from the SON on key community organization boards (this information should be available in the accreditation reports of the school).
- Review the university board of directors to determine if there are any nurse members.
- Review public relations documents from the institution to determine the emphasis given to the nursing unit.
- Ask key faculty members how they are recognized for their accomplishments within the university or among community groups.

STRATEGY #4

Understanding the Benefits ("Perks") of the Position

Salary is only one component of the benefits provided by employment, even though it receives the most attention from prospective faculty. For example, a lower salary at an institution that invests 10% of your gross salary (up to the maximum allowed) into a retirement fund may be more beneficial in the long run (if you plan to stay at the institution for an extended period) than a higher salary from an institution that invests 5%. Although you may think that tuition reimbursement benefits for dependents are not important to you and your future, it does not hurt to know the policy in relation to your tuition support. You may decide to take a foreign language class to prepare yourself for future cross-cultural research. If your health benefits are covered by your partner's employer, you might be able to negotiate other benefits. Most institutions like to offer a standard benefit package; sometimes the benefits are more flexible. If you do not ask about benefits, you will be offered the standard minimum package. You may also want to ask about the flexibility of certain other components of the benefits.

Let's assume that each faculty member receives $300 per year to cover expenses associated with attendance at professional meetings. You need to know if the policy is an annual "use it or lose it" policy or if you can carry over the $300 from one year to the next. Or if you agree to assist with some of the coverage of the school's booth, could some of your travel expenses beyond the $300 be covered? Generally, the more questions you ask about benefits, the better you will be able to evaluate the true benefits that accompany the position.

Tips

- Obtain as much written information as possible about the standard benefit package of the institution. Standard inclusions are health insurance and contributions to some level of retirement plan. There are, however, many other benefits that can be included or optional, such as life insurance for you and your dependents, child and family care benefits, tuition support for you and your dependents, etc. The variation from one school to another is great, so you will need to make a careful comparison.
- Obtain as much information as possible about the benefits that are offered by the SON that may be above and beyond those included in the standard university benefit package.
- Ask as many questions as you can regarding benefits and perks; take notes, and go back for a second visit with someone in the benefits office.
- Ask your colleagues who have faculty positions at other comparable institutions what is included in their perks.
- Create a list of "must have" benefits and ones that are "nice but not necessary."
- Determine if the absence of any benefit will be a determining factor in declining a position.
- Identify the time frame when certain benefits become available; e.g., some tuition benefits become available only after you have been in a position for a certain number of years.

Understanding the Expectations Above and Beyond the Position Description

It is often the case that once you are in the faculty role, you find out that there are some things you were not told about the expectations for all faculty members. Or worse yet, that the expectations for faculty are unclear or unrealistic. You ask yourself why it wasn't possible to know about some of these expectations early in the position or in the interview process. As is the case with almost everything about a new role, the more you know beforehand, the better prepared you are to address the issues or to adjust to the new expectations.

One of the worst things that can happen to you is to find out that you have made the wrong decision about a position because you did not thoroughly understand the expectations in your new role. If this happens because of your own lack of assessment, learn from the experience, reevaluate the pros and cons of the position, and determine if it is advantageous to stay. If the position is untenable because the expectations have changed, because they are other than what was originally described, or because they have become unrealistic due to changes in personnel or the overall situation, consider whether it is wise to stay in the position. This will require you to do a thorough assessment of the situation and to determine the best course of action. Discussions with mentors can be particularly useful at this time.

Tips

- Inquire about any other information that is relevant to the position or to your future evaluation.
- Ask faculty members who are at your rank whether there were any surprises they experienced in the first year of their position.
- Ask the person who will be your immediate supervisor what expectations he/she might have beyond what is formally expressed in the written documentation.

- Try to assess the potential changes that could lead to changes in expectations, e.g., a substantial increase in the number of students entering the program without an increase in numbers of faculty.
- Evaluate the pros and cons of staying in a position in which the expectations are unclear, unrealistic, or constantly changing.
- Seek advice from mentors or experienced faculty colleagues.
- Evaluate the activities that are within your control, and manage those well.

STRATEGY #6

Providing Just Enough Personal Information in the Interview

Most people talk too much in a job interview and provide too much personal information that is not relevant to the position. Sometimes it may seem as if this is the best way to relate to the person conducting the interview, but usually it is just due to anxiety. Keep in mind that it is always better to discuss aspects of one's professional life rather than one's personal life. Try to deflect questions about your personal life with answers that are related to your professional life and goals.

Prior to a job interview it is most useful to consider how you will respond to inquiries about personal aspects of your life. It may be helpful to role-play the interview with a friend or colleague. Consider all the possible questions you may be asked by others and what information you would like to provide. If you want to keep your personal life private, practice your responses to any potentially personal questions that you think you may be asked. At the same time, you do not want to appear distant and lacking in social graces. For example, you may be invited to a meal where conversation about personal matters may seem casual. Remember, there is no such thing as casual conversation in a job interview. Everything you say will be repeated, even if it is said in the hallway and not in a formal interview session. Be cautious and constantly on guard. (See Appendix F.)

- Carefully consider the components of your personal life that you want to discuss in a job interview.
- Role-play with a friend or colleague so that you have some practice responding to difficult personal questions.
- Maintain a positive, upbeat attitude and conversational tone throughout the interview.
- Avoid talking about other professional colleagues, especially about their personal lives.
- Consider ways to reduce your stress while in the interview process, and practice some stress-reducing exercises beforehand, as oftentimes individuals under stress will talk too much just to fill the silent pauses in the conversation.

STRATEGY #7

Knowing About Imminent Changes in Leadership

Often the retirement plans of key members of the administration are known but not officially announced. If you just ask someone in the system, it is easy enough to find out. It is particularly important for new faculty members to find out the retirement plans of the key academic administrator, in most cases the dean of the SON. Much of the tone of the SON, including the specific goals, is dependent on the dean of nursing rather than the faculty. This is in contrast to other departments in universities, so it is important to understand.

It is less likely that you will be able to predict the resignation of key individuals when the choice is based on their recruitment to another, more prestigious, position, or when the resignation is not their choice. Forced changes in leadership are particularly problematic within the institution as they are often signals of other systemic problems. It will be important for you to reassess the situation and to determine if the projected changes are central to your functioning as a faculty member. If it is still possible for you to achieve your short-term goals while the transition occurs, then there is no need for you to be concerned about your own status within the organization.

Remember that transitions in key leadership positions are very common and that the institutional goals and processes governed by the faculty, i.e., the curricula, are the most important aspect of your work.

- Ask questions about expected turnover, including plans for retirement, of key administrators.
- Assess the overall stability of the system, particularly in relation to key administrators remaining in their positions.
- Evaluate what effect a major change in administration would have on your position.
- Review the process for evaluation of administrative staff and determine to what extent you want to participate in that evaluation.
- Determine the effect of key retirements on the position you hold.
- Determine if the time frame for the planned retirement of the key academic leader is consistent with your time frame or if it is irrelevant.

STRATEGY #8

Portraying Your Attitude and Motivation

An attitude and motivation check is an important part of the initial self-assessment that a candidate should complete. No one wants to hire a faculty member with a negative attitude and a lack of motivation. If asked, prospective employers say that a positive attitude is one of the most critical attributes of an employee. Clear your mind of other distractions, and focus on the interview when it occurs. For example, if you are worried about extraneous concerns during the interview and therefore do not give the person your full attention, your behavior may cause the interviewer to misjudge your attitude.

You will most likely be asked about your motivation for seeking the particular position. Thus, it is important that you give this some serious prior thought. You will certainly be judged partially on your motivation for seeking the position and your ability to concisely put it into words. It is wise to consider motivation for a particular position in relation to your overall 1- and 5-year career goals.

Tips

- Ensure your attitude before proceeding to an interview is positive.
- Do not add any negative comments to your responses; there is no reason to be negative regarding others or former employment experiences.
- Identify your motivational goals based on your future career goals.
- Identify resources that might help you develop a more positive attitude, such as any number of motivational books.
- Consider finding a career coach to help you with your overall career planning, including attitude development.
- Ask your colleagues to give you honest feedback about how your attitude comes across to them.
- Consider a role-playing session with a trusted colleague; videotape or audiotape the session so that you can assess your intonation and attitude in conversation.

STRATEGY #9

Evaluating Job Security Issues

Many nontenure positions have 1-year term contracts, and others have 5-year terms. It is important to understand the possibilities within the SON. If there is a multiyear contract, ask whether the salary remains the same for the term of the contract or if there are opportunities for annual salary increases.

Job security may be as related to the local shortage of faculty as to any other factor. If there is a large number of individuals in your geographic area prepared at the same academic level as you are, then there is more need to be concerned about job security.

It is key to evaluate your short- and long-term goals in relation to job security issues. If you are viewed as having changed positions too frequently, e.g., annually, then this may affect the next position offer. Consider the term of the nontenure contract, and negotiate for a multiyear contract with an opportunity for annual salary increases if you are interested in remaining in an academic position. Then be certain to successfully accomplish and/or exceed the expectations for nontenured faculty for advancement and promotion.

- Inquire about the contract terms for nontenured faculty.
- Evaluate the criteria used for reappointment of nontenured faculty.
- Plan your short- and long-term goals so as to successfully achieve and/or exceed the expectations for faculty at your rank.
- Discuss issues of job security with mentors, senior faculty, and administrators at the school.

STRATEGY #10

Effective Salary Negotiation Skills

Salary negotiation is difficult for most of us, as we feel inadequate and inexperienced in the process. As with many other components of the process of finding a faculty position, the general rule of thumb is that the more information you have, the better prepared you will be to negotiate wisely.

Fortunately, there are guides that can help you understand the level of salary you should request. Many public universities are required to publish the salary levels of faculty members, so this is an important resource to obtain. These lists are published on the university Web sites or in the campus newspapers; they should be easily accessible through a computer search of the institution. In addition, the American Association of Colleges of Nursing publishes an annual guide to faculty salaries by level of institution as well as by faculty rank. Other faculty at the institution, or comparable institutions, are often willing to share information about their salaries. Of course, it is important to use discretion in doing so.

The most important thing is to know the range of salary that you will be offered rather than the individual salary that is tied to a position. Depending on the number of candidates for a position and your credentials, you may or may not have the "upper hand" in the negotiation process. You should recognize all the factors that will influence the salary negotiation and understand that your goal is to create a "win-win" outcome. (See Appendix O.)

Tips

- Review and evaluate published guides for salary.
- Consider your base salary in relation to these guides, not additional salary that might be provided for extra summer teaching or other activities.
- Decide your desired salary, how much you are willing to negotiate, and your minimum salary requirement.
- Consider other elements of the benefits package within your overall negotiations, and remember that some benefits may be negotiable. For example, you might be able to negotiate for some support for traveling to professional meetings or conferences. Thus, instead of this funding coming from your own resources, it would be paid by the institution. If you negotiate for other benefits, be certain to have these detailed in writing as administrators change.
- Consult with others about comparable salaries at the institution, in other departments, within the same school, and in comparable universities in the same geographical location.
- Consider how important salary is to you. For example, you may be willing to accept a somewhat lower salary for the chance to work with the key person in your field who could serve as a mentor for your future scholarship.

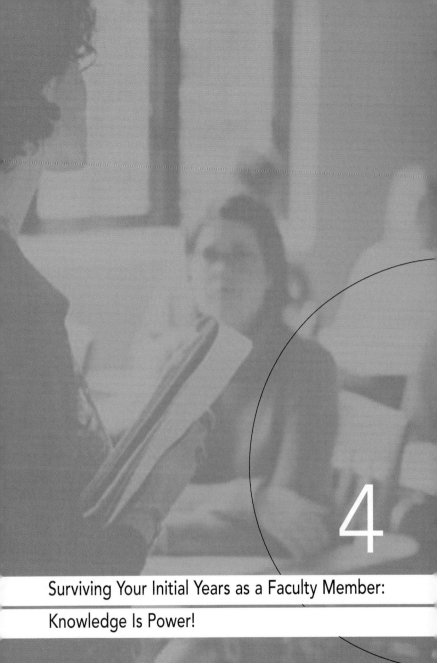

4

Surviving Your Initial Years as a Faculty Member:

Knowledge Is Power!

STRATEGY #1

Developing Networking Skills

Networking is a skill that is very important in the academic world. You will want to develop networks of colleagues within your institution and a broader network among colleagues throughout the world. Most often, networking relationships extend beyond the boundaries of institutions, and with the use of electronic communication, academic nursing networks now extend globally. The professional networks that you develop should be understood as career networks, targeted to your area of scholarship. Networking involves creating win-win relationships so that all members benefit. In contacting others to create a networking relationship, be certain to indicate that there is benefit to them as well as to you. For example, you might be able to help researchers obtain access to a new population, or you might invite them to do a presentation in your community. Even if these activities are not of interest to them in the immediate future, the fact that you have offered them something is important.

Never underestimate the power of networking. You never know who knows whom and how it will be beneficial to your future career. Those who are very experienced at networking and those who take it very seriously keep data-based files on all of their contacts so that they can retrieve the information for some future purpose. The most important principle might be to treat all colleagues as potential future employers, as you never really know how successful anyone will be. It is possible that some of your current students may end up being your future bosses.

In addition to networking, it is important to develop colleagues wherever you go, building your base of collegial relationships as your career progresses. It is wonderful to have colleagues throughout the globe. Academic nursing covers a small world, one that is becoming smaller each year.

- Develop your networking skills. (See Appendix U.)
- Develop a skill for remembering the names of all those you meet.

- Build your skills at developing collegial relationships, finding a mutual benefit in collaboration with colleagues.
- Develop an understanding of the nature of partnership for teaching, research, and publication.
- Practice thinking positively about creating win-win situations.
- Always consider the other person's career development goals as well as your own.

A guide to networking is provided in Appendix U.

STRATEGY #2

Accepting the Perfect Position for You

It's a buyer's market in the search for faculty, meaning you will have lots of choices of positions if you have some flexibility. There is a faculty shortage and one that is expected to increase in the next two decades (see Appendix X). The first job offer you receive may not be the best one for you to accept. If you have done the comparative analysis recommended above, you may not have to "jump" to accept the first offer. If you are anxious that you may not find a position that meets your time requirements, it will be more likely that you will jump too soon at the first offer. Also, those who do not consider all aspects of the job search may be more likely to say "yes" too quickly. Even if you are told that there are other qualified candidates waiting to hear if you are going to accept the position and/or that the institution needs to know immediately for other reasons, it is always better to wait a few days and evaluate the overall standing of your job search.

While you are waiting, you should review your academic career goals and consider how this position will help you achieve those goals. Weigh the positive and negative aspects of the position, and consider how close it is to the ideal position that you have in mind. Consider what would happen if you were to decide not to accept the position for another 2-4 weeks and whether you could tolerate losing the position if it were to be offered to someone else.

- Identify a clear time frame for the components of your job search, working backward from the time of desired new (or first) employment.
- Obtain information about the time frame for each position that you are considering, including the start date and the date when the selection of the candidate is to occur.
- Communicate your time frame to those who are interviewing you for positions or those who are the key decision-makers in the search process.
- If your time frame does not match that of the institution, consider whether you are willing to change your time frame or whether to exclude that position from the search.
- Decide whether you want to have a flexible or fixed time frame.
- Identify what factors might lead you to alter your time frame.

STRATEGY #3

Meeting the Key Persons With Whom You Will Be Working

In the interview process, you may not have met all of the key individuals with whom you will be working if you accept the position. For example, you might have met the course coordinator but not the faculty members with whom you will be teaching. Perhaps you met the undergraduate program director but not the course coordinator in your clinical area or the dean of the SON. If you have not met all the key individuals during the interview process, be sure you do so before accepting the position, especially those who will participate at some level in your future evaluations.

Be assured that a request for a second set of interviews and/or meetings is not unusual and should not be considered in poor form. This job decision is very important to your career development, and you need to have as much information as possible. You need to consider all aspects of your proposed working environment. Those colleagues with whom you will be working day to day are extremely important to your success.

Tips

- Study the organizational chart to identify key individuals within the system, and determine how the position you are applying for fits within the structure and whom you need to meet.
- Request meetings as soon as possible with the key individuals, and be flexible about the meeting dates and time, fitting your schedule to those of the individuals with whom you are requesting meetings.
- If one of the key positions is vacant, ask if you can participate in the selection of the individual for that position.
- If the request for meeting the key individuals is denied, consider this as part of the overall information about the system, and determine if you want to work in a system that is closed to such requests.
- Consider whether you will accept the position if you do not have the opportunity to meet with these key individuals.

STRATEGY #4

Serving on Committees

In addition to teaching and scholarship responsibilities, all faculty members are expected to serve on committees at the school, university, or community level. Expectations about the extent of involvement in university, professional, and community service vary, depending on the nature of the institution and the rank of the faculty member. Generally, those of higher rank are expected to be more involved at all levels. Although it is important to do one's share of the work that needs to be done, school and university committees and professional service responsibilities can interfere with the core activities of teaching and scholarship. Ascertain the expectations for new faculty members (independent of rank), and maintain your involvement at the minimal level at least for the first 1-2 years.

Once you have developed an understanding of the expectations for your service on school and university committees, select the ones that you are most interested in and those that are most closely related to your position, and communicate your interest in serving on these committees to the chair of your department or program. For example, if you teach in the undergraduate program, you may want to serve on the admissions committee for that program. If your area of expertise is mental health, you may want to serve on the student services committee. Try to coordinate your faculty service responsibilities so that they add to your overall professional portfolio. You may want to volunteer for a new committee, e.g., bylaws, because you want to learn more about the faculty governance at your institution.

Tips

- Ascertain the minimum expectations for school, university, professional, and community service and the way in which such service factors into criteria for advancement within the system
- Be selective in choosing committees for involvement; do not take on major responsibilities that will interfere with your teaching and scholarly productivity.
- Ask the advice of your mentors when deciding which committees to join.
- Select activities that are interesting for you as well as ones that will add to your overall faculty and professional credentials and that are consistent with your career goals.

STRATEGY #5

Understanding Unionization

Many faculty members in nursing have little awareness of the reasons for unionization or the details of the union contract. The first question you should ask is whether there is a union contract for faculty and, if so, who is included. Some contracts cover only full-time tenure-track faculty. If there is a union contract for faculty, obtain a copy, and read it carefully. Find out the history of contract negotiations and the key players both at the university and the school levels. Generally, the presence of a union for faculty members at a university or school is not a key factor that should influence whether or not you accept a position, but it is important that as a new faculty member you understand all aspects of the faculty organization and the relationship to the administration.

It also is important to know if there is a union contract for other members of the university staff, e.g., clerical or maintenance workers. These individuals will be needed by you at some time in your employment and it is important to know the relationship that they have within the overall structure. This is something that is not critical for you to know before accepting a position and certainly will be less relevant if you are in a part time or clinical position as you will not need their services as frequently. Also, there is often one person in the school who manages human resources for both faculty and staff. You should know who that person is and what the job responsibilities are for this person.

- Early in your employment, find out if there have been any discussions about faculty unionization.
- Develop an understanding of faculty governance for the school, including issues of academic freedom.
- If there is a union, review all formal documents; know the details of the organization that represents the faculty.
- Ask questions about the formal documents if they are not clear.
- Meet with key representatives of the faculty to discuss the faculty organization, whether or not there is a union representing them.

STRATEGY #6

Prioritizing Parenting Responsibilities While on the Job

Parenting is an extremely important role. But parenting should not be done "on the job," and it should not interfere with the responsibilities that one has assumed in a teaching position.

Yet, many academic institutions have very tolerant policies regarding parental leave. And they are very tolerant of the day-to-day needs of families. It is not unusual for teachers to have their children in the office when it is a grade school day off. However, before assuming that that is acceptable, find out the policy at your particular institution. When in doubt, it is always best to inquire. And do not take advantage of the system's flexibility and tolerance. Err on the side of caution.

Also, it is important that you communicate your personal emergency plan to the key authorities at both the school your children attend and your place of employment. Make certain that the key administrators know how to contact you in an emergency and that you know how to advise your children if you have an emergency at work. With parenting responsibilities, it is always smart to have contingency plans in place should any situation arise.

Tips

- Know the formal policies regarding parental leave at your institution.
- Ask others about the norms for behavior, and when in doubt inquire at the human resources department.
- Develop your own level of comfort with the dual responsibilities of parent and teacher.
- Seek support from others who have similar role conflicts and/or expectations.
- Make friends with other families so they can provide a support system in times of need.
- Obtain as much outside help as you can afford.
- Forget about domestic and parenting perfection.
- Create a plan for your children so they know how to reach you in emergencies.

STRATEGY #7

Understanding the Benefits of Technology

Technology has become an integral part of the academic world. Many courses are Web-enhanced, and many schools have moved to Web-based courses of one variety or another. If you are not conversant in the latest applications of technology to both academic nursing and health care, an introductory course in nursing informatics with particular attention to applications in nursing education would be useful before entering or reentering the academic world. The content available for classroom instruction has greatly expanded with the use of the Internet. In addition, there are a number of software programs that are most useful in expanding access to new information and enhancing teaching.

While there is more variation in the application of technology in the clinical arena, depending on the size and location of the clinical facility, overall there has been significant change in the past decade. A reorientation might be required for those who are returning to clinical teaching, even after a brief hiatus, particularly as your students will be required to use the new technology in nursing practice.

It is a continuing challenge to remain current in technology. One suggestion is to gather a group of colleagues at your college or university who are interested in continuing education and plan regular sessions where you share experiences using the new technology in the classroom or in the clinical arena. New faculty will find this a great learning experience. You also could use this as a model for students who want to stay current; they can develop study groups focused on technology application experience. Nowadays, there is usually at least one computer wizard in the class who is happy to provide instruction to other students.

Tips

- Determine what the norms are for the application of technology in the courses you will be teaching and clinical facilities you will be using.
- Assess your own knowledge and skills in the use of technology in education.
- Assess your own knowledge and skills in the use of technology in clinical practice.
- Acquire knowledge and skills that may be lacking in the application of technology to your teaching and clinical practice.

- Identify the experts in your academic setting, both within the SON and throughout the campus.
- Learn from others who have expertise in this area, whether colleagues on the faculty or students in your class who have well-developed computer skills.
- Plan to include at least one new technology application each semester in order to gradually enhance your learning and expertise.

STRATEGY #8

Identifying Resources for Faculty Development

Faculty members need to know what resources exist both within the school and in the larger university to assist with their individual and collective faculty development. Find out this information early in your employment.

Faculty development from within the SON might consist of access to research and teaching development resources, continuing education at the place of employment, financial support for continuing education that exists off-site, and/or financial support for travel to key professional meetings. In addition, there may be a formal process of mentoring that exists to help faculty members toward promotion and tenure. Some SONs retain consultants for faculty development in the areas of editing manuscripts and advising on scholarship. Knowing about the resources available is the first step in accessing them.

In addition to the resources available within the SON, it is important to know if there are any of these same resources supported at the university level. This is information that is usually not available on the Web site but rather comes from informed questions directed to key administrators.

 Tips

- Create a list of resources that would be helpful to meet your immediate 1-year and 5-year career goals.
- List the resources within the SON.

- Identify resources within the university.
- Compare resources at other comparable SONs. You might be able to find out this information by asking key questions when you attend local, regional, or national nursing education meetings.
- Determine how important these resources are to you and how you might help your department consider them for future new faculty members (such as yourself).
- If the resources are not available within the school or university, determine how you might access them individually to meet your own professional goals.

STRATEGY #9

Understanding the School's Practice and/or Incentive Plan

In the past decade several SONs have developed practice and/or incentive plans for faculty. These plans have different goals; they are not all like the practice plans that are part of the long history of schools of medicine. Yet, some SONs have chosen to become part of the medical practice plans in the schools of medicine. Some SONs have chosen to model their practice plans after the medical practice plans. Others are more inclusive, with other income generation included. For example, any nursing-related income-generating activity could be included in the practice plan. Some plans also include consultation and royalty income. More general incentive plans have been designed to reward faculty for securing grants for the school. Funds are allocated to either faculty salary or benefits (travel, professional organization fees) based on a percentage of the overall grant funds. Even though practice and incentive plans are not yet commonplace in SONs, it is important that you be knowledgeable about the ones that do exist. (See Appendix Q.)

- Inquire about existing practice and/or incentive plans within the school.

- Review the history of the development of the plan and the relationship to the mission of the school.
- Review the plans thoroughly to determine how they will affect your compensation.
- Discuss the plan with the key administrator responsible for implementing the plan.
- Determine how the plan influences your work and professional goals.
- Determine how the plan is related to the criteria on which you will be evaluated.
- If the school does not have a practice plan, ask about future plans to develop incentive plans or faculty practice plans.

STRATEGY #10

Understanding the Criteria for Promotion for Tenure-Track vs. Nontenure-Track Faculty

It is important to understand the differences in criteria for advancement between the two levels of faculty, particularly if you have a choice about which type of position to accept. This information should be easily available in the formal documents, but you may also wish to gather some informal information from senior faculty and key administrators.

Requirements for nontenure-track faculty vary from institution to institution and often within the schools of the same university. Have as much information as possible about the expectations before accepting a nontenure-track position. Most often the form of scholarship that is expected of nontenured faculty is teaching or expertise in clinical practice, without the requirement for formal research. Publications are expected of nontenured faculty, so this should be understood.

Some nontenured faculty members are content to remain at the beginning ranks within the academic institution and thus do not concern themselves with publishing and advances in scholarship. In this case your career goals may not include progression within the academic system. The important thing is to match your career goals with the type of position, and plan accordingly.

- Review formal documents for promotion for nontenure-track faculty.
- Inquire about the history and the current experience with nontenure tracks within the SON.
- Identify key persons who could provide informal information about the nontenure track and the differences between tenure-track and nontenure-track positions.
- Match your choice of type of position with your career goals.
- If you are uncertain about your long-term career goals, discuss your options with key members of the administration of the school or with mentors.

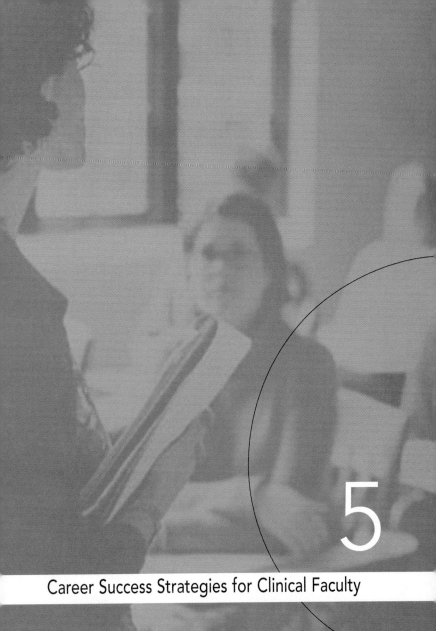

5

Career Success Strategies for Clinical Faculty

Striking the Perfect Balance of Clinical Practice and Teaching Skills

Overemphasis on maintaining clinical practice skills or neglecting clinical practice to enhance teaching skills is problematic because both skill sets are needed for effective clinical teaching. While maintaining certification is important and requires a set number of practice hours, such requirements must be balanced with developing teaching skills that will enhance your teaching. At the same time, your teaching will benefit from continued clinical practice in which your skills and knowledge are up to date.

If you do not have the background in one of these two key areas, you should consider how this will affect your progress in a faculty position and how it is related to your overall career goals. You may wish to discuss this with a mentor or with the program administrator. If you do not have the clinical skills, the students that you are teaching will be aware of this lack of expertise. The same is true for the lack of teaching skills. Both skill sets are learned through experience and formal preparation. Thus, once you determine the need, it will be possible for you to develop the skills.

Tips

- Consider your career goals for balance in maintaining expertise in clinical practice and developing teaching skills.
- Intersperse clinical practice with teaching, and balance the number of conferences or continuing education attended in both areas.
- Consider online learning to enhance knowledge/skills in either area as available.
- Do not become discouraged if you are not expert in both areas; developing teaching and/or clinical skills takes time and practice.
- Become knowledgeable about the research on nursing education, as there are new developments in this area.
- Consider studying for teacher certification, at the same time maintaining certification in your clinical area.

Knowing the Value of Clinical Teaching Skills

Entering into the clinical area with a group of students without any previous knowledge or skills in teaching is never a good idea. Some general knowledge of the principles of adult learning and effective clinical teaching experience are necessary. Students quickly recognize someone who is unprepared.

It is important to understand the clinical arena in which you will be working and have good clinical skills as well as to develop good clinical teaching skills. These skills have not often been included in advanced practice nursing programs, so you may not be the only faculty member who needs to develop and/or enhance clinical teaching skills.

Many clinicians think that if they can practice expertly, then they can teach others to practice. This is not always the case. Some of the learning depends on the background, learning styles, and learning experiences of the students. Some of the success also depends on the manner in which the clinical content is presented. There are ways to develop expertise in clinical teaching.

- Find a mentor who can advise you as you develop clinical teaching skills.
- Read the basic nursing education textbooks, particularly those focused on curriculum and instruction, evaluation, and preceptor skills.
- Review nursing education journals periodically as they often contain useful teaching tips.
- Suggest a faculty development session focused on clinical teaching. It may be led by a member of the current faculty, or you may invite a national expert if there is financial support.
- Ask your students for daily feedback about your clinical teaching so that you can learn what is effective and enhances their learning.
- If there are teaching experts on your campus or a center for teaching, consult with experts who are there to provide the service to faculty.

Ensuring You Get a Thorough Orientation to the Clinical Site

Different clinical units often have very different protocols for patient care. Failure to get a thorough orientation to the clinical site can have disastrous implications. You will spend excessive amounts of students' clinical time trying to figure out how things are done, which impedes learning and creates chaos. In addition, students and hospital staff are likely to become annoyed.

There are also differences among units in the same clinical sites. Some of the procedures are based on the expertise and/or preferences of the nurse manager, but clinical policies may be missing or not well developed. Not all of the procedures you need to know will be in writing. It should not be the case that as clinical instructor you assume that you are visitors on the unit or in the hospital. You are assuming partial responsibility for patient care.

If, as a clinical instructor, you determine that the clinical environment is unsafe for student learning, your responsibility is to report this to the program and course director. Safety issues can arise due to inadequate staffing, to unsafe practices, or to inconsistency in the policies and procedures. Students should not be learning or practicing in unsafe clinical environments.

Tips

- Arrange for at least a basic orientation to the clinical site before students begin their experience.
- Be familiar with the policies and procedures of the unit you will be working on. This includes reviewing policy and procedure manuals and other materials that familiarize you with the site.
- Identify a resource person that can be available to you for questions or concerns.
- Report any unsafe practice conditions or environments to the program chairs.
- Help students understand factors that influence safety in clinical settings.

Closely Monitoring All Students on the Clinical Site

Students have different ability levels and cannot always accurately appraise their own abilities. Faculty members who do not closely monitor students in the clinical setting may find that students have given inappropriate medications, treatments, or procedures. Students may have been overconfident or misunderstood what was ordered for the patient's care.

There are many different protocols for monitoring student behavior in the clinical setting. It is extremely important that clinical faculty members understand that as part of their responsibility they must know what the students know and permit them to function accordingly. The faculty member assumes some of the legal responsibility for the students' clinical behavior, and mistakes can be very costly. Patient safety is a new mantra for hospitals and other clinical agencies; there are many opportunities for system failures or personal mistakes that lead to patient injuries.

 Tips

• Check in with students frequently throughout the clinical day.
• Require students to check in with you within the first 2 hours of clinic to present their plan of care for the day. Understanding their individual patient care plans can help you assess students' thinking and ensure that they are practicing safely. However, this does not mean that other issues will not come up that require the students to make judgments about patient care.
• Students who are having difficulty should be monitored more closely and should be assisted to develop an appropriate plan of care for their patient(s).
• Insist on the student-faculty ratio that is best for student learning and that ensures a safe practice environment. This may vary from one clinical facility to another and clinical specialty, but generally an 8:1 or 10:1 ratio is considered the maximum.

• Take appropriate action to see that students who do not practice safely are asked to leave the clinical environment.

STRATEGY #5
Ensuring Clinical Competence

Clinical practice changes rapidly. Do not assume that because you taught something previously that you are still current. When feasible, try to avoid teaching in clinical areas outside your area of expertise. Lack of knowledge can be detrimental to patient care and can hamper student learning.

With the current shortage of nurse faculty, the demands to teach in areas that are not familiar to you will increase. It is very important that you are clear about your teaching assignment and that you are confident of your own expertise in that area. If you are not, bring the issue to the attention of the program director. The clinical agency will expect that the faculty members have expertise in the areas of assignment.

• Prior to teaching in a new area or one that you have not practiced in recently, review some basic nursing texts in the content area to give yourself a refresher.
• Reviewing the summaries or key points sections of a general textbook (like one the students will use in class) can also be helpful.
• Talk to nurses on the unit where you will be working to gather information about specific clinical protocols.
• Attend some of the lecture classes with the students for areas that you identify as weaknesses.
• Negotiate with your faculty chair or dean to teach in areas that are strengths and in which you have the most experience.
• When there is enough advance notice, attend continuing education programs to refresh or gain knowledge.
• Consider online continuing education opportunities.
• Refuse to teach in clinical areas in which you judge your expertise to be inadequate.

Understanding the Faculty Practice Plan

Familiarity with your school/college's faculty practice plan is critical. Individuals who do not ask the right questions prior to employment might find significant drawbacks in a faculty practice plan that does not fit well with their individual goals. Many practice plans set limits in terms of practice, including hours, and income that must come back to the school from individual faculty practice.

Not understanding the practice plan requirements may present difficulties to your career advancement. You will be expected to be knowledgeable about and to abide by all of the stipulations in the contract. It will also be likely that you will sign a formal contract that includes mention of compensation as related to the practice plan. Know the restrictions on your practice as well as the benefits to having the practice plan in place. (See Appendix Q.)

Tips

- Carefully review the institution's faculty practice plan prior to accepting employment.
- If a copy of the faculty practice plan is not included in materials sent to you prior to your interview, it may be accessible via the school's Web site. It is wise to review this plan before the interview. This will facilitate your being prepared for discussion with administration and other faculty and will give you enough background knowledge to ask meaningful questions during the interview.
- In many settings, all new faculty members are required to join the faculty practice plan.
- Carefully analyze if the faculty practice plan is going to meet your personal goals and financial needs.
- It may be useful to compare faculty practice plans among differing institutions to get an idea of what strengths each offers.

Becoming Involved With the Core Activities of the School and University

In many settings, clinical faculty members are only minimally involved with activities of the school and university. Lack of involvement reflects negatively on the individual and prohibits the faculty member's voice from being heard in important decisions related to the faculty role. Although clinical faculty may have fewer voting rights within the university, members can still have a significant impact if they choose to participate at the school/college level.

As a clinical faculty member, it is important that you view your role as integral to the school's mission and goals, for without quality clinical instruction the program would not survive. Very often, clinical faculty members are not oriented to the overall programs and activities, or even to the policies and procedures for clinical supervision of students. Some of the responsibility for this oversight belongs to the school, but it is also important for the individual clinical faculty member to take the initiative to become knowledgeable and involved.

Tips

- Find an area of school governance that is of interest to you, and get involved in that area.
- Review the mission and goals of the school and the documents outlining responsibility of clinical faculty members.
- It is not to your advantage to take on unessential tasks that are not of interest to you. There may be some things required of you that you are not interested in doing. However, for those activities that are extra, chose an area that interests you more.
- Talk to other faculty to determine strengths and weaknesses of certain roles to find the best match.
- Work with a colleague on a role, when possible/feasible, to make it more tolerable.
- Agree to take on a role in the interim to see if it is a good fit before making a long-term commitment.

• Select committee roles that expand your horizons into a new area; in doing so you are less likely to become bored.

STRATEGY #8

Understandng the Importance of Including Families in Care

Families are an integral part of nearly every patient's life. Neglecting to include them in the plan of care can have negative consequences. For example, in many cultures the family is consulted before any significant decisions are made. Therefore, it is important for the nurse to understand that these members of the family need to be included. Nursing students often need to have a role model to integrate this skill into their practice.

Including families in the patient's care also gives another person exposure to information about disease processes and discharge planning. The process of inclusion will help the families, the students, and the patients, as there will be an opportunity for all to learn from each other. If you have not had experiences in institutions where family members are encouraged to become involved in patient care, it will be important to become oriented to this model of care so that you can teach it to the students.

• When discussing with students their initial plan for care, be sure to ask them how they plan to include the family.
• Integrate discussions about family into post-conference and have students attend continuing education or other presentations about working with families, when feasible.
• Have students address families in nursing care plans and other required course work.
• Become knowledgeable about models of family-centered patient care.
• Serve as a role model for students, helping them to understand the value of involving family members as part of the health-care team.

Understanding Legal Implications

Significant legal liability is involved when working in a nursing role caring for other persons. When you are covering students in their practice, additional legal responsibilities are assumed because the students are working under your license. It is important that you be aware of these considerations in order to protect yourself as well as the students. You need a working knowledge of what procedures are within the student role and what policies and practices apply to the agency. For example, students may not be permitted to give blood or start IV lines.

The clinical faculty member also should be clear about the liability coverage that is in place. Different models are used in different academic institutions. Some institutions self-insure students and faculty, and others have contracts with insurance companies. You should be certain what is expected of you regarding professional liability insurance, especially in high-risk areas such as maternity and pediatrics. You also should be familiar with the level and type of coverage required of the students under your clinical supervision, whether they are basic nonlicensed students, or postlicensure registered nurses, or advanced practice students. At the same time, different clinical agencies will also have different expectations for these levels of students. In the case of legal matters, you can never have too much information.

- Become familiar with the policies of the hospital, unit, and university before clinical instruction begins.
- Review the legal requirements of each institution.
- Review your professional liability insurance policy carefully, and determine if the coverage is sufficient, especially if it covers your clinical supervision role.
- Make certain that students have the appropriate insurance coverage.

- Make certain that students understand the legal aspects of their role.
- Talk to other faculty members who have taught at the site to learn helpful hints
- Be familiar with your state's Nurse Practice Act.

STRATEGY #10

Selecting Appropriate Clinical Assignments

Inappropriate clinical assignments can occur in several ways. First, the faculty member may not have a good understanding of an individual student's clinical skills and inadvertently assign a patient that the student has little ability to care for. In some instances, the student may be at fault for inadequate preparation. In either case, the faculty member must assess that the student has some background knowledge to care for the particular patient assigned.

The faculty member may not be aware of what content has been covered in class so far. Students should not be expected to care for patients about whom they have not had any classroom content. The faculty member should keep track of the content covered in lecture and assign students accordingly.

Inappropriate clinical assignments can also stem from shortages of staff on the units or in the facilities. It is important for the clinical faculty member to understand responsibilities for monitoring and reporting any unsafe working conditions and to make certain that these conditions do not interfere with student learning. This problem is expected to increase as the shortage of nurses increases. Students should not be used as replacements for nurses employed by the facility.

- Keep track of what the students are learning in lecture and what content previous courses have covered.

- Carefully examine students' knowledge while in the clinical setting and post-conference to get a good idea for their substantive strengths and weaknesses.
- Monitor the staff-patient ratios as they might affect student learning and clinical assignment of patients.
- Report unsafe conditions because they introduce liability issues and affect student learning.

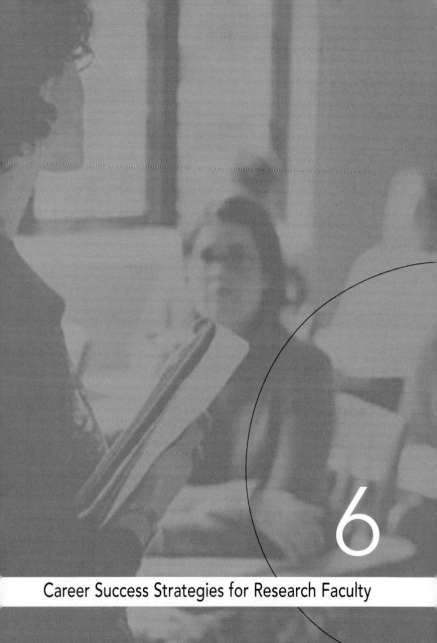

6

Career Success Strategies for Research Faculty

Matching Your Research With Your Place of Employment

A poor research match at your place of employment can have disastrous effects on ultimate success. While completion of the doctoral degree ensures that one is minimally competent to do research, mentorship and additional experience is necessary for success. If resources at your place of employment are not available to help you succeed, you won't. Faculty colleagues who do not understand your research ideas, methodology, or clinical area may have difficulty helping you develop strong research proposals and secure funding. Additionally, you may have difficulty finding collaborators.

In addition to content and methodological match, it is important to find an institution that has a similar research philosophy. Mismatch in terms of the amount of research you are expected to accomplish can also hamper your career success. For example, if you go to an institution that focuses extensively on teaching, you may not have support for your research plans. On the other hand, if you only want to dabble in research, a Carnegie I institution (see Appendix P) would not be a good match, as the expectation here is that a large portion of your time is devoted to research.

- A good research match at one's place of employment can facilitate individual research development.
- A good match includes people with clinical, methodological, and research ideas similar to your own.
- Access to individuals with the experience and expertise you need will facilitate your development as a researcher and will help you meet your research goals. These individuals can provide specific advice and critique of your work and can give you an idea of what might be funded in your particular interest area.
- Experienced individuals will know what resources are available on campus to facilitate your work and can often

put you in touch with colleagues who share similar interests. Resources are more likely to be supported by the individual college or university if there are many people using them.

- Finding a good fit in terms of the amount of time devoted to research is also critical to career success. The easiest way to get a sense of research expectations and the resources available is to talk to people, both formally and informally, who work at and in conjunction with the institution. This can be done through networking, formal interviews, reviewing the Web site, and reviewing materials produced by the institution.
- When possible, contacting individuals who are no longer involved with the university can be equally helpful. Understanding why people leave can also help you assess the workplace.

STRATEGY #2

Developing an Effective Mentorship

Effective mentorship is key to success in any position. It is even more critical for research. As discussed previously, individuals must have adequate research mentorship to be successful in research. Inadequate or ineffective mentorship can leave the new faculty member struggling with how to accomplish research goals. Struggles can be very minor, from, for example, locating Institutional Review Boards forms online, to severe, such as struggling with the appropriate research design to answer a research question. Whereas minor struggles mostly amount to wasted time and inconvenience, major struggles lead to inappropriate research ideas and research proposals, lack of funding, and lost opportunities for learning, building skills, and gaining experience. Over time, inadequate or inappropriate mentorship can lead to multiple rejected proposals, a negative reputation for the faculty member, and perhaps a bad reputation for the college or university. In addition, it is likely that a tenure-track faculty member may not be reappointed or may be denied tenure. Resources of the college and university are wasted on a poor product or are invested in a faculty member who is unlikely to be successful. For the faculty, time spent in a role that does not provide satisfaction, motivation, or increased knowledge can lead to poor mental health and lost future job opportunities.

 Tips

- Find a senior colleague who can "show you the ropes" of the institution, both in terms of getting things done and in research development.
- Develop relationships with others who can critique your work and will provide opportunities for you to critique theirs.
- Let colleagues know you want to be apprised of available opportunities for career development (e.g., practice reviewing grants, presentations, other contacts). (See Appendix M.)
- Join groups on campus with similar interests that can facilitate your career development (e.g., research centers, informal groups, work groups).
- Remember that you can never have too many mentors.
- If someone is not helpful to you or not available when you need assistance, ask for help elsewhere.
- Do not take advice that you are given personally or get defensive.

STRATEGY #3

Developing an Appropriate Plan to Secure Funding

Success in research takes careful planning. Identify a research program early in your academic career, and identify potential increasing levels of support. Beginning with pilot support is a key step. Those who make funding decisions like to see a pattern of previous funding, as the best investment is in those who have demonstrated success. Once you develop your plan to secure funding, it will be easier to evaluate your research productivity against this plan. You should develop a method for self-review of your progress toward funding.

A haphazard approach to research planning and funding will not likely result in success. A proposal that is "thrown together" at the last minute in order to make a deadline probably will not put your best showing forward and be funded. Repeated poor efforts may lead to a poor reputation among funding agencies and potentially negative publicity for the college/university. Over time, negativity can have multiple influences and stifle career success.

A major step for securing early funding is having a feasible plan in place to complete the proposed idea; equally important is the ability to articulate what the next research steps will be and how initial funding will contribute to knowledge development. Failure to explicitly identify these issues will likely endanger funding.

Tips

- It is easier to get funding once you have been funded. Therefore, focus initial efforts on securing some funding, even if it is small, so you can begin to establish a track record.
- Pick a research topic that is important to someone in addition to you. Others must understand the problem that needs to be investigated if they are going to invest in your work.
- Once you have developed the idea for investigation, think about the long-term sustainability of the idea and if the next steps are feasible for you to pursue. This can help you decide if there is long-term potential in your idea.
- Write your research plan down to refer to at a later date. It may help generate new ideas and stimulate thinking. It may also help to remind you of what your previous thinking was.
- Build on what you began with your dissertation work only if the topic can sustain your future research career/trajectory and is fundable.
- Research funding rules in the job search process. Ideally, you had funding for your dissertation, or you have funding to take with you.
- If you do not have funding to take with you to your first research position, make sure you have a solid plan to get funding.

Developing a Strong Research Team

Great care must be taken in putting together a research team. Your research team should consist of individuals who can add to your knowledge and expertise in conducting the research. For example, if it is not evident from your scholarly credentials, i.e., publications and previous research experience, that you have the statistical expertise to conduct your study, then you should be certain to have someone with statistical background and expertise on your team. In your proposal you will be expected to explain how each team member will contribute to the research project.

Research team members will expect to contribute to the overall scholarship, including participation in publications. Discuss the expectations at the time that the team is forming, and clarify the issues of authorship with all involved. If the research idea is primarily yours, then you should retain first authorship on publications.

A research team that consists of too many (or all) junior investigators will not be judged strongly by reviewers and will have less chance of being funded. Also, if one of the team members does not have strength (including both publications and previous grant funding) in relevant portions of the research project, the project is not likely to be funded. An essential aspect of a competitive research proposal is that it have scientific merit (significance of the research and the methodology to conduct the study). The research team members must complement each other and have demonstrated expertise relating to the proposed research.

Tips

- It tends to be easier to receive funding if you have someone on your team who has been funded.
- When forming your research team, keep in mind the complementary skills of the members as well as the need for collaboration. Select individuals who work well together.

- Clearly outline the responsibilities of the team members, including expectations for authorship on publications. Do not leave this to chance or deal with publication authorship informally.
- Identify and formalize expectations for order of authorship on all planned articles as a result of the research, keeping in mind the general rule in nursing that the order of authorship is based on amount of contribution to the article, with the person who contributed most being the first author.
- An individual with current funding shows the reviewers that a certain level of expertise has been achieved. This strengthens your team.
- Don't try to do it alone. Multidisciplinary and interdisciplinary research is expected.
- Team members should have complementary skill sets.
- A history of working well together bodes well for funding success.

STRATEGY #5

Preparing Adequately for the Faculty Research Role

Entering into a tenure-track position as a new PhD graduate can be a significant challenge. Depending on the quality of your doctoral experience and dissertation and the expectations of the school, a significant gap may exist in knowledge/skills and what is expected of you on the job. Carnegie I Research–classified schools will have significant expectations for research productivity from faculty. For example, you may be expected to obtain extramural research grant funding before progressing in your position or before being promoted to another faculty level. If you did not attend a doctoral program at this level of school, merging into a faculty role at a Carnegie I Research institution will be difficult, if not impossible, without additional training/experience. Although there are mechanisms in place to prevent the hiring of individuals not qualified for certain positions, as a candidate it is equally your responsibility to evaluate the position carefully.

Be certain that you understand the expectations for scholarship of both the university and the school, and plan your short-term goals accordingly to meet these expectations. If you do not meet the expectations during the first year or two, then every successive year will be more difficult to "catch up." If it is not clear how you should balance your time in order to meet the requirements, then seek guidance from mentors and senior faculty and administrators. Keep in mind that your research and scholarship are the most important components for research-intensive universities.

Many top-ranked schools have institutionally funded postdoctoral programs. These are federally funded programs (often by the National Institute of Nursing Research [NINR] at NIH) to which individuals can apply. Ideally, these programs have multiple scholars and faculty experts to enhance the learning experience. In addition, postdoctoral programs may have monthly research sessions and additional resources to promote research skills and experiences. You may also apply for individual postdoctoral funding through NINR if you can establish that you have a good mentor, research plan, and adequate resources available to conduct the proposed work. However, the process is lengthier when applying for funding as an individual.

- Postdoctoral education/training is a viable way to gain valuable research skills and experiences with a senior researcher who has interests similar to yours.
- If you take part in a postdoctoral program, make sure the mentor match is excellent and that you are completely confident that your experience will be a positive one and meet your research development needs.

STRATEGY #6

Obtaining Writing Experience

Writing is an essential part of the faculty role. Dissemination of research findings and the ability to communicate clearly are necessary job components. Lack of experience in writing and communication during graduate work is a costly mistake. Many students who simply commute to class and do not become involved in the work of their school during graduate and/or doctoral preparation are particularly at risk for inadequate writing abilities. Missing the opportunity to publish with distinguished faculty to help guide you through the process and to help you develop your own ideas and writing style can be major impairments to career growth beyond the degree program. When inadequate experience is gained during the educational process, significant amounts of time are used up in writing and revising, among many other activities competing for attention.

Often the best teacher for developing writing skills is experience. The more you write, the more comfortable you become with the process, including the successes and failures. For most faculty members, writing does not come naturally; it is a skill that has to be practiced. Do not shy away from practice opportunities, including the potential opportunity to publish with other faculty members.

Tips

- Make yourself available to gain needed experiences during doctoral work.
- Participate in writing projects with faculty whenever possible.
- Generate your own ideas, and with the assistance of a trusted colleague develop the idea into a manuscript.
- When appropriate and timely, turn classroom (course-work) assignments into manuscripts that can be submitted for publication and/or presentation.
- Learn the basics of successful writing, including taking time to write daily rather than saving up your writing and expecting to accomplish it in major blocks of time.
- Attend a workshop on scholarly writing. Many journal editors present these workshops at conferences and professional meetings.

- Develop your writing skills by completing a continuing education program; these are offered both online and through conferences.
- Celebrate your successes in writing, sharing your published articles with mentors and professional colleagues.
- Encourage your school to celebrate the successes of all faculty members who have published by creating a special showcase or bulletin board.

STRATEGY #7

Using Time Between Employment Opportunities Wisely

Even though it may be distressing to be between jobs for a while, use the time wisely to accomplish goals that will facilitate future job opportunities. Many people will not do any work except look for work. This is a mistake, because much can be accomplished between semesters or after the completion of doctoral work.

The best way to use your time is to identify some specific goals that can be matched to the time frame. For example, if you have only a month between positions, do not attempt to write two articles, as this will be setting yourself up for failure. Set goals that are realistic to accomplish, and stick to them. Organize your time so that some part of each day is devoted to your professional development. Even if you set aside only 1 hour per day, you will be surprised how much you will accomplish.

Also use your time to learn new skills that might be useful in your career. For example, you may wish to enroll in a continuing education program focused on applying technology in clinical practice or one focused on faculty development strategies. There are many programs offered throughout the country, in your local community, and through self-study programs on the Internet. It is very important that between positions you return to your assessment of your strengths and weaknesses and develop a plan for addressing some of those weaknesses, even if the greatest weakness is procrastination.

101

Tips

- Publish your dissertation as soon as possible. Ideally, your manuscript should be in review before you begin your new position.
- Use time to put research and manuscript ideas on paper and, time permitting, develop those ideas more fully.
- Any work that can be accomplished prior to an official academic appointment gives you a head start.
- Remember that new positions always come with many things of a "task" nature to accomplish (e.g., getting keys, obtaining parking, etc.), so time spent on important tasks now will be well appreciated later.
- Develop a research and/or publication plan that can be shared with potential employers. It shows that you are organized and have developed some ideas that you will continue to work on once employment commences. It shows others you are ambitious and interested in getting things done.
- A well-developed research plan will help you to assess "fit" with an organization and what resources you might need to be successful.
- Attend local, regional, and national conferences to network with others and learn about potential job opportunities. Conferences will also help to keep your knowledge current.

STRATEGY #8

Selecting the Best Journal for Publication

Occasionally, individuals will submit a research manuscript to the first journal that comes to mind, just to get it published. It is more effective to publish in the best journal possible. A manuscript that is published someplace easy might not reach the intended audience and may not get the attention it deserves or communicate the research findings to the intended audience. Good research that is published in a poor journal can also be ignored or be inaccessible if libraries do not subscribe to the journal. Author reputation may also suffer.

In determining your publication goals, it is best to review all the potential targeted journals and to ascertain both the audience they reach and the specifics of the manuscript processing. Then you will want to match your goals with the goals of a journal. For example, if the content of your manuscript would be most useful to clinicians, then you want to select a clinical journal that has a wide circulation. If your research is focused on nursing education, then your targeted audience includes nurse educators. This will lead you to journal selection. Mentors can help you determine where to submit your manuscripts for potential publication, and you should not hesitate to ask their advice. (See Appendix V.)

Tips

- Publish your dissertation in the best journal possible.
- Generally, journals that have "research" in the title or that focus primarily on research are regarded most highly.
- Target your manuscript submission to a journal where it will receive a good deal of publicity through a large subscriber base. Journals that are a member benefit for professional organizations may be useful for this purpose.
- To help target the best journal, determine who will benefit from the research. Consider whether a research journal or a clinical journal is a better fit.
- Check the journals impact factor via the ISI Web site at http://www.isinet.com
- Be sure to follow all the journal's guidelines before submitting the manuscript.
- Learn how to "sell" your research by the introductory wording of your topic. You should understand that you must convince the editors and reviewers that your scholarship makes a substantial contribution to the literature. Address the questions "So what?" and "Who cares?" in describing your research results.

Using Available Resources to Accomplish Your Goals

Career success can be enhanced if you tap into all available resources. There are many people who can help you in your career development, and you should not shy away from using the resources available, including both the institutional services and the people within the institution. For example, many universities have centers for teaching to assist faculty to develop and use new teaching techniques. You should do a thorough assessment of the resources available on your campus and determine the best way to access these resources. Failure to have others read your work or to utilize available university resources can be detrimental.

Most helpful to you will be other faculty. Sometimes senior faculty members are more available than you think, and all you have to do is ask them for assistance. Before doing so, it is most helpful if you have assessed your own learning needs and career development needs. You should decide if you want advice about overall publishing or if you have a particular manuscript that you would like them to review. In asking someone for assistance, it is helpful to let them know your time frame as well. For example, if you want their feedback within a 2-week period, let them know that, and they will be able to decide if they can meet the expectation. Lack of contact with key members of the faculty and/or one's dissertation committee can mean trouble in the manuscript and research proposal development process.

Tips

- Utilize your dissertation committee and other trusted experienced colleagues to assist you with the publication process.
- Identify faculty members at your new place of employment who can assist you with publications and other career development activities.
- Have others review your work. A good read by someone with content expertise as well as someone without can greatly

improve your writing. The content expert reads for accuracy, and the nonexpert reads for clarity of writing and your ability to communicate the message intended.

- Investigate what resources are offered by your university or local library that may be of assistance to you: for example, writing centers and/or workshops, faculty experts, Internet access, print and electronic media, and many others.
- Form a support group with other colleagues so you can keep each other focused on important career goals.

STRATEGY #10

Putting Your Dissertation Horror Stories Behind You

Although the doctoral and dissertation processes are wrought with difficulty, dwelling on negative experiences accomplishes nothing. Repeating your horror stories to your colleagues, students, or potential employers does not put you in a positive light. The dissertation is designed as a learning experience. Thus, you should focus on "lessons learned" and use these lessons positively to help colleagues who might be going through the process. In addition, even your negative experiences can provide growth experiences in teaching, as you can use these to help guide your mentoring of others in their research and career development processes.

Use your experiences to assist others in the process of developing their own work. Create a list of the things you would do differently, and use those ideas in both your teaching of others and your future research supervision.

- Put your negative dissertation experiences behind you and move on.
- If you need to write it down and burn it, do it!
- Remember the learning that was embedded in the experience and build on the learning rather than dwell on the specifics that may have been negative.

105

- Use your "character building experience" to create positive experiences for others.

STRATEGY #11

Using Time Wisely on the Tenure Track

With the many opportunities available for intellectual stimulation at most university campuses, new faculty members often become overwhelmed and thus fall behind in their research and scholarship activities. Overbooking your schedule limits how much time you have available to work on projects directly related to the criteria for tenure and promotion. Inadequate progress in research and scholarship is likely to result in termination.

Most of us gravitate toward the work that leads to immediate satisfaction and that which is most familiar to us and therefore easiest to accomplish. For a new faculty member, this often does not include the work that is most central to promotion and tenure. It is important to create a list of goals and a time frame toward tenure that will help you to structure your choice of activities. For the pretenure-track faculty member, each new activity should be weighed against the criteria for tenure. If the opportunity is not directly related to your progress toward tenure, then you should pass it up. There will be plenty of other opportunities that come your way once you have achieved tenure.

In order to achieve tenure, it is very important that you know the explicit requirements within your institution and that you know the process that you should follow. Each institution is different, and you cannot assume that what has applied in previous employment situations will apply in your current situation. Ask as many questions as you can so that you are clear and thus can use your time wisely. (See Appendix N.)

- Carefully select the work you agree to do. Only take on projects that contribute to meeting the guidelines for tenure and promotion. Generally, these activities include securing research funding through proposal submission, working on other research-related activities, scholarship, teaching, and service to the profession.

- Be clear on the relative weight that is given to each tenure criterion. For example, faculty members are often expected to engage in professional service, but not at the expense of scholarship. Rather, the professional service is viewed as "icing on the cake." It is never a substitute for scholarship.
- Know your institution's tenure and promotion guidelines, and make your choices carefully.
- Save documentation related to the activities you are doing that support your case for tenure and promotion, including evaluations, thank-you notes, papers, proposals, etc.
- Organize your documentation so that it will be easy to assemble; be sure to update your curriculum vitae routinely (perhaps once per year or once per semester) so that you have an ongoing record of your accomplishments.

References

Monday, D. (2004). Interview dressing tips. Available: http://www.top-career resumes.com/interview-dressing-tips.html Accessed April 19, 2005.

Vault.com. (2005). Interviewing. Available: http://www.vault.com Accessed April 18, 2005.

Key References

Books

Davis, B. G. (1993). Tools for Teaching. San Francisco: Jossey-Bass.

Huber, M. T. (2004). Balancing Acts: The Scholarship of Teaching and Learning in Academic Careers. Washington, DC: American Association for Higher Education and The Carnegie Foundation for the Advancement of Teaching.

Journals

Chronicle of Higher Education
http://www.chronicle.com

Journal of Nursing Education
http://www.journalofnursingeducation.com/about.asp

Journal of Professional Nursing
http://www.aacn.nche.edu/Publications/jpn.htm

Nurse Educator
http://www.nursingcenter.com/library

Nursing Education Perspectives
http://www.nln.org/nlnjournal/index.htm

Key Web Sites

American Association for Higher Education
http://www.aahe.org

American Association of Colleges of Nursing (AACN)
http://www.aacn.nche.edu

American Association of University Professors (AAUP)
http://www.aaup.org

American Nurses Credentialing Center (ANCC)
http://www.ana.org/ancc/

Carnegie Foundation for the Advancement of Teaching
http://www.carnegiefoundation.org

Chronicle of Higher Education
http://www.chronicle.com

Higher Education.com
http://www.highered.com

National Certification Corporation (NCC)
http://www.nccnet.org

National Institute for Nursing Research (NINR)
http://www.nih.gov/ninr

National League for Nursing (NLN)
http://www.nln.org

Nurses for a Healthier Tomorrow Career Information
http://www.nursesource.org

The Princeton Review
http://www.princetonreview.com

The University of Michigan Division of Student Affairs Career Center (reference letter information)
http://www.ccp.umich.edu/students/refletter/writingguide/writingletter.html

University of Waterloo Career Development Manual
http://www.cdm.uwaterloo.ca/step1.asp

Vault (general career information)
http://www.vault.com

Professional Organizations Relevant to Faculty

American Association for Higher Education (AAHE)
American Association of Colleges of Nursing (AACN)
American Association of University Professors (AAUP)
National League for Nursing (NLN)

Faculty Certification

Certification for faculty can be obtained in a clinical specialty area or in teaching. Both options are discussed below.

Clinical Practice Certification

Clinical practice certification can be done at the registered nurse (RN) or advanced practice level. The American Nurses Credentialing Center (ANCC) is the predominant body that certifies RNs. ANCC is the credentialing arm of the American Nurses Association (ANA). Detailed information about the certification process can be found on the Web site at http://www.ana.org/ancc/ Requirements for certification vary, based on the examination to which the candidate is applying. General requirements include academic degrees, practice hours, and continuing education. Certification is granted for 5 years and is renewable through continuing education.

The National Certification Corporation (NCC) is a nonprofit organization that provides certification for the women's health and maternal child specialties of practice. NCC is completely separate from ANCC and therefore has independent criteria for candidates applying for the examination. However, the processes are similar. Certification is for 3 years. Detailed information can be found on the Web site http://www.nccnet.org

Teaching Certification

The National League for Nursing (NLN) is in the process of developing a certification examination for nurse educators. The NLN is anticipating pilot test development at a future summit, with regular administration to follow shortly afterwards.

Rankings of Schools/Colleges of Nursing*

U. S. News & World Report periodically evaluates graduate schools based on several criteria. Below are the rankings for graduate nursing programs in 2003.

Adult Nurse Practitioner

1. University of Pennsylvania
2. University of Washington
3. University of California at San Francisco

Adult Medical-Surgical Clinical Nurse Specialist

1. University of Washington
2. University of California at San Francisco
3. University of Pennsylvania

Community/Public Health Clinical Nurse Specialist

1. University of Washington
2. Johns Hopkins University
3. University of North Carolina at Chapel Hill

Nursing (Master's)

1. University of Washington
2. University of California at San Francisco
3. University of Michigan at Ann Arbor
4. University of Pennsylvania

*Additional information and rankings can be found at http://www.usnews.com
   National Institute of Nursing Research (NINR) funding rankings of research intensive schools of nursing can be found at http://grants1.nih.gov/grants/award/trends/dhenrsg03.htm

Nurse-Midwifery

1. Oregon Health and Science University
2. University of Pennsylvania
3. University of Illinois at Chicago
4. University of Michigan at Ann Arbor
5. University of Minnesota at Twin Cities
6. University of New Mexico

Nursing Anesthesia

1. Virginia Commonwealth University
2. U. S. Army Graduate Program in Nurse Anesthesia
3. Navy Nurse Corps
4. Rush University

Nursing Service Administration

1. University of Iowa
2. University of Pennsylvania
3. University of Washington
4. University of North Carolina at Chapel Hill

Psychiatric/Mental Health Clinical Nurse Specialist

1. University of Washington
2. University of Pennsylvania
3. University of California at San Francisco

Interview Guide*

- Put yourself in the mind of the interviewer and critically critique yourself, including how you look or present yourself.
- Expect questions that address organization, attention to detail, people skills, how you think, and weaknesses.
- Review the job description and any corresponding information prior to the interview.
- Review the university and school/college Web sites.
- Expect some behavioral-type questions—those that address what you did or would do in a given situation.
- Make sure you follow up with a thank-you note following the interview.

*Information from vault.com

Key Components of a Reference Letter*

- Reference letters serve as a way for students to market themselves to potential employers or educational institutions.
- Write letters only for students you know well enough to provide adequate detail and objectivity.
- Letters that compare the applicant with his/her peers are generally considered more useful.
- Include information on the student's communication skills, writing ability, resourcefulness, analytical ability, ability to work independently, ability to complete projects in a timely manner, patience and attention to detail, leadership abilities, clinical skills (if appropriate), and teamwork.
- Be honest. Those requesting the letter will appreciate your honesty.
- Limit the letter to one or two pages.
- Indicate how you know the student.
- Frame your comments to the student's goal (e.g., admission to graduate school, job application).
- Keep comments objective.
- Support your comments with specific examples.
- Obtain the student's permission to include information regarding any extenuating circumstances.
- Use official letterhead stationery, and type the letter.

*From the University of Michigan Division of Student Affairs Career Center: http://www.cpp.umich.edu/students/refletter/writingguide/priorwriting.html

Components of a Teaching Portfolio or Dossier

Include items that are most relevant to your work or that you wish to highlight:

- Syllabi
- Outstanding student work
- Letters or other comments from students
- Innovative teaching in the forms of strategies, assignments, or courses
- Publications related to the scholarship of teaching
- Grants for educational research
- Teaching awards or outstanding citations
- Faculty and course evaluations

Guidelines for Student Advising

- Advising is a personal and individualized process.
- Advising forms a critical link between the student and the institution.
- Advisors do more than help students pick courses; they nurture, encourage, support, and inform.
- Advisors give students general career advice.
- Advisement promotes learning and intellectual, physical, and personal development.
- Advising may involve many people and departments on campus (e.g., home [major] department, disability services, athletics, honors college, etc.).
- Students need clear and concise explanations of the curriculum and needed courses.
- A review of what the student has left to complete should be assessed routinely at each appointment.
- Information on study skills, career options, academic policies, graduate or professional school admissions, and how to access university services may be needed by students.
- Be prepared for all possible information requests, and have ready access to information to facilitate productive advisement appointments.
- Web addresses are helpful for providing students with information you do not have.

Self-Assessment to Determine Career Goals

The University of Waterloo has a comprehensive self-assessment tool on its Web site at http://www.cdm.uwaterloo.ca/step1.asp. This Web site features a series of assessment tools and activities to assist with career development choices. The self-assessment focuses on pride experiences, personality, values, skills, interests, knowledge, self-employment suitability, and integrating what you have learned. The Web site is easy to follow and allows printing of tools.

Another self-assessment tool can be found on The Princeton Review Web page at http://www.princetonreview.com/cte/quiz/career_quiz1.asp. This career quiz estimates personal interests and usual style by having you select the best option between two choices. There are 24 questions.

Guide for Developing
a Curriculum Vitae (CV)

- Academic CVs require all relevant content to be included so that one may trace the development of your career.
- Include your education, past and current employment, publications, presentations, awards received, grant funding received, and any outside committees or task forces you were involved with.
- Be comprehensive but organized.
- Ensure your CV is easy to read and follow.
- Use headings for new categories (e.g., publications, presentations).
- Bold type can be used sparingly throughout to help separate sections or highlight achievements.
- Include your full name, contact information (including e-mail), and any licenses or certification.

Appendix L

Guide to Dressing for Success

Appropriate dress for a job interview is crucial for success. And the importance of appropriate dress does not end once the job is offered or accepted. In general, one should dress conservatively for a job interview, and this pattern should continue after employment begins. It is always better to be more conservatively than too casually dressed. Over time, you will develop an idea for what is considered appropriate dress at your institution. Some faculty members are expected to wear suits everyday, whereas others are permitted to dress more casually, with suits donned for specific events (e.g., important meetings, faculty candidate interviews, etc.). Generally, dark colors, such as navy, black, or gray, are best. Dress shoes should be in good condition, and generally dark colors with a low-to-medium heel are best. Hair and nails should be clean and well manicured. Avoid perfumes or aftershave. "Noisy" items such as bracelets, earrings, or other jewelry should also be avoided. Body piercings should be removed and tattoos covered.

Key Tips on How to Find a Mentor for Career Development

- Identify individuals who possess skills or experiences you wish to gain.
- Mentors can be identified from the university faculty and the broader community.
- Attend functions on campus and in the community to meet potential mentors.
- Be involved in various groups that will expand your access to potential mentors as well as valuable experiences. These groups can include research projects, task groups, community groups, hobbies, and religious organizations.
- Reviewing the literature and attending conferences is another way to become familiar with the work of individuals who might make worthwhile mentors.
- When you identify someone you think might be valuable as a mentor, interact with him/her. This will help you establish if you have similar personalities and working styles as well as common interests. Interaction also has the potential to lead to opportunities for collaboration.
- Seek the advice of senior faculty and others for ideas about mentors and events that might be beneficial to attend.
- Regular follow-up with a mentor can facilitate opportunities and continued mentorship.

Criteria for Appointment and Tenure Review: What You Should Know

There are criteria specific to each faculty rank. It is important to note that adjunct and clinical faculty may be appointed at any rank of the university based on credentials. In most universities and SONs, the order of appointment is normally: instructor, assistant professor, associate professor, professor (full professor). The criteria that will be used to review your position will vary from school to school. Remember that most universities have formal policies regarding process for review. These documents should be readily available to you in a printed or electronic format and are generally published in the bylaws of the faculty in the faculty handbook.

In regard to tenure review, find out the specific criteria for your school or university. It will be important to learn when the "clock starts" for tenure consideration. The pretenure time frame is usually 7–9 years. It may be that there is a formal comprehensive review process midway in the pretenure period. Find out if your previous teaching experiences will count toward tenure. Do years at another university count, or is tenure at this institution solely based on time spent here? Remember that it may or may not be possible to change from the nontenure to the tenure track. In addition, find out if there are circumstances that "stop the clock" in terms of achieving tenure. It is common for the granting of tenure to mean an automatic promotion to associate professor.

It will be most important regarding your tenure or appointment review to find out the weight at your institution given to:

• Meeting expectations in terms of the number of courses taught per year
• Teaching evaluations

123

- Student course evaluations
- Demonstrating teaching innovation
- Number of publications within a certain time frame
- First authorship
- Quantity vs. quality of scholarship
- Data-based publications vs. other types
- Extramural research
- Principal investigator on grants
- A comprehensive self-evaluation comprising teaching, publication, and professional service documentation and any awards, leadership positions, or special citations.

Salary Guidelines

Nurses for a Healthier Tomorrow advocacy group reports that in 2002 nurse educators who were employed full-time with 9-month appointments earned between $25,000 and $185,000. The average salary for nurse educators with a doctoral degree was $61,000. Faculty with a master's degree earned an average of $49,000.

The American Association of Colleges of Nursing (AACN) provides comprehensive salary data based on a variety of factors including administrators, medians, academic and calendar year, rank, and undergraduate/graduate. A hard copy of the report can be ordered through the Web site http://www.aacn.nche.edu

For public institutions with state employees, salary information is often considered public knowledge. This information can be accessed through individual state Web pages.

The Chronicle of Higher Education provides national faculty salary data that are available online for subscribers.

The American Association of University Professors (AAUP) has published a report titled "Inequities Persist for Women and Non-tenure Track Faculty: The Annual Report on the Economic Status of the Professor 2004–05," which is available at www.aaup.org

Carnegie Classification of Higher Education Institutions

- Doctoral/Research Universities—Extensive: These institutions award 50 or more doctoral degrees per year across at least 15 disciplines.
- Doctoral/Research Universities—Intensive: These institutions award at least 10 doctoral degrees per year across 3 or more disciplines or at least 20 doctoral degrees per year overall.
- Master's Colleges and Universities I: These institutions award 40 or more master's degrees annually across 3 or more disciplines.
- Master's Colleges and Universities II: These institutions award 20 or more master's degrees annually in 1 or more disciplines.
- Baccalaureate Colleges—Liberal Arts: These institutions are primarily undergraduate colleges with major emphasis on baccalaureate degree programs. They award at least half of their baccalaureate degrees in the liberal arts.
- Baccalaureate Colleges—General
- Baccalaureate/Associate's Colleges
- Associate's Colleges
- Specialized Institutions—Theological seminaries and other specialized faith-related institutions
- Specialized Institutions—Medical schools and medical centers
- Specialized Institutions—Other separate health professions schools
- Specialized Institutions—Schools of engineering and technology
- Specialized Institutions—Schools of business and management
- Specialized Institutions—Schools of art, music, and design
- Specialized Institutions—Schools of law
- Specialized Institutions—Teachers colleges
- Specialized Institutions—Other specialized institutions
- Tribal Colleges and Universities

More detail, including the 2005 Revision of the Carnegie Classification System and the classification of specific institutions can be found at http://www.carnegiefoundation.org

Key Elements of a Faculty Practice Plan

Purpose

To serve as a model for expert nursing practice

To provide opportunity for precepting students

To provide opportunities for faculty and graduate student research

To provide financial incentive for faculty who engage in practice

To serve as a model site for translational research

Key Components

- The faculty plan represents a formal contract between the faculty member and the "practice plan," and the clinical agency and the "practice plan."
- Any policy and/or procedural changes must be approved by the "practice plan" and the SON administration.
- Percentage of time devoted to practice may vary each contract year, and usually a minimum percentage is specified.
- Faculty practice plan may be required or optional for full time faculty.
- Faculty benefits through the "practice plan" are specified in writing, including compensation, travel support, research funding, and conference fees.

Activities That Most Often Comprise the Plan

Clinical practice/patient care

Consultation

Research (extramurally funded)

Training and education seminars

Strategic planning consultation

Lectures and presentations with honoraria attached
Legal consulting, including expert witness services

Other Important Issues

Malpractice insurance coverage
Benefit formula (e.g., is the income from the plan included in the
    retirement allocation from the university)
Vacations, sick time, and coverage
Bonus calculation formula; schedule for fee payments
Billing practices
Regulatory and credentialing issues
Relationship to promotion and tenure evaluations
Interdisciplinary collaboration and contractual relationship with
    consulting physicians

Contractual Agreements With Clinical Agencies for Student Placement

I. General Agreement

A. Cooperation in the provision of clinical experiences for undergraduate and/or graduate students enrolled in the School of Nursing.

B. Agreement will be in effect for 1 year from the date, and will automatically be extended from year to year for an indefinite period unless one of the parties notifies the other party in writing sixty (60) days prior to the end of any yearly period that the contract is not to be renewed for the following year.

C. Agreement is not assignable but is binding on the successors of the parties. This agreement is not a third-party beneficiary contract and confers no rights upon any students or employees of the parties.

D. Parties agree not to discriminate on the basis of race, religion, age, sex, color, disability, sexual orientation, national or ethnic origin, political affiliation, or veteran status.

II. University Responsibilities

A. Faculty member selection and assignment for clinical instruction; will notify Agency of faculty members responsible (names and qualifications) and will provide names and academic status information on all students to have clinical experience at the Agency at the beginning of each semester.

B. Cooperatively with Agency will arrange for appropriate orientation of faculty members and students.

C. Will make preceptor arrangements in accordance with Agency policies.

D. Responsible for validating that students and faculty have current professional/personal liability insurance.

E. Responsible for determining that faculty members and students are in satisfactory health and will provide health records as necessary.

F. Will assure that faculty and students comply with any health requirements of the Agency, e.g., drug screening, etc.

III. Agency Responsibilities

A. Will provide, without cost to the university and its students, clinical resources and facilities for use in their educational experiences.

B. May, after discussion with the University, terminate clinical privileges of any student whose performance is unsatisfactory or whose behavior presents a danger to the interests of the Agency or its patients.

C. The students will actively participate in the care of patients in accordance with the guidelines set forth by the Agency, provided however that such students shall at all times be supervised by appropriate Agency personnel. The Agency retains ultimate responsibility for the nursing care of all patients, including those assigned to students. The Agency agrees to carry professional liability insurance coverage, sufficient to meet claims brought within any applicable period of limitation, with respect to its patient care activities and to name the University and its participating faculty, students, officers, and employees as additional insureds. The Agency will provide a copy of the insurance certificate to University upon request.

D. The Agency understands that information received regarding students participating in clinical training is subject to the provisions of the Family Educational Rights and Privacy Act and agrees to use such information only for the purpose for which it was disclosed and not to make it available to any third party without first obtaining the student's consent. Health records will be destroyed following the completion of the student's experience.

Formal signatures of University and Agency Administrative Officers are usually required.

Appendix

S

Components of Student Course Evaluations and Teaching Evaluations

Most institutions have a standard form/format that is used for course and teacher evaluations. Many institutions now conduct evaluations online. The following items are typically included in course and teaching evaluations:

- How well students' learning needs were met
- Teaching effectiveness
- Comprehensiveness of content
- Enthusiasm for and knowledge of the subject matter
- Classroom environment
- Use of technology/course management software (e.g., BlackBoard, Coursetools)

Key Components of a Course Syllabus

- Faculty of record
- Faculty contact information (including e-mail address)
- Course number and title
- Number of credits
- Placement in the curriculum
- Course description and overview
- Time, location, and schedule of class meetings
- Course objectives
- Assignments
- Grading for assignments
- Grading tool(s)
- Expectations for student behavior
- Teaching methods
- Learning resources
- Required and recommended course materials (books and other resources)
- Attendance or other relevant policies

Guide to Networking

Networking is a form of communication that can help build and maintain professional relationships. It is a systematic way of building relationships with others in your professional area. It is also about building a community of professionals around yourself to enhance your career. Those in your network can provide valuable advice on career decisions and development.

The Basic Steps of Networking

- Know yourself, including strengths and limitations.
- Identify professional goals.
- Identify others in your area who may be able to help you.
- Read everything that known academics have written in your area of interest.
- Do any additional background research required on your topic of interest.
- Identify commonalities that lie between your area of interest and those of others in the field with whom you wish to connect.

Approaching the Person With Whom You Wish to Network

If possible, let your publications be your introduction. If you have not yet published, your resume will serve as a second-best introduction. Briefly explain your career goals. Then tell the person why you want to network with him or her. Be sincere and flattering. Comment on the other's work and contribution to the field and why it is important to you. However, be brief and concise in all of your communications, whether at a conference or through written communication/e-mail.

Next, make sure that you follow up your contact and that the other person knows how to reach you by e-mail, mail, and/or phone. For example, schedule a face-to-face meeting with her/him at the next professional conference. Maintain contact following your meeting in person. Ask for advice about your career goals and your immediate scholarship goals and projects.

The Negative Connotations of Networking

- Networking is knowing the right people and using them to career advantage.
- Networking is playing politics.
- Networking is playing the career game.
- Networking interferes with real work.
- Networking is time-consuming.

Always be genuine and sincere in your relationship with those in your network, but always maintain a positive response and positive relationships. Before contacting anyone for networking purposes, consider how you can reciprocate, e.g., you might be able to have the more senior person invited as a consultant where you work. Try to keep a level of objectivity about your network. Take a step back, and write down your networking goals for a specified period. For example, each year review where you are in developing new contacts in your professional life, and set new goals for networking. Make sure to work with a diverse group of individuals, as long as you have identified the professional commonalities. This will help you avoid potential conflict or competition with others in the network.

Tips for Building a Publication Record

- Start small.
- Submit manuscripts to journals or other avenues where you are likely to have early success.
- Find a writing mentor.
- Work with experienced writers to learn the process.
- Get to know as many editors as possible. Use your mentor to help you meet these key individuals.
- Share the work.
- Write about topics that interest you and that will be of interest to others.
- Respond to "call for manuscripts" notices, as journals may be short of papers, increasing your odds of acceptance and earlier actual publication.

American Association of University Professors Tenure Rules

Recommended Institutional Regulations on Academic Freedom and Tenure

The Recommended Institutional Regulations on Academic Freedom and Tenure *set forth, in language suitable for use by an institution of higher education, rules which derive from the chief provisions and interpretations of the 1940* Statement of Principles on Academic Freedom and Tenure *and of the 1958* Statement on Procedural Standards in Faculty Dismissal Proceedings. *The* Recommended Institutional Regulations *were first formulated by the Committee on Academic Freedom and Tenure (Committee A) in 1957. A revised and expanded text, approved by Committee A in 1968, reflected the development of Association standards and procedures. Texts with further revisions were approved by Committee A in 1972, in 1976, in 1982, in 1990, and in 1999.*

The current text is based upon the Association's continuing experience in evaluating regulations actually in force at particular institutions. It is also based upon further definition of the standards and procedures of the Association over the years. The Association will be glad to assist in interpretation of the regulations or to consult about their incorporation in, or adaptation to, the rules of a particular college or university.

Foreword

These regulations are designed to enable the [named institution] to protect academic freedom and tenure and to ensure academic due process. The principles implicit in these regulations are for the benefit of all who are involved with or are affected by the policies and programs of the institution. A college or university is a marketplace of ideas, and it cannot fulfill its purposes of transmitting, evaluating, and extending knowledge if it requires conformity with any orthodoxy of content and method. In the words of the United States Supreme Court, "Teachers and students must always remain free to inquire, to study and to evaluate, to gain new maturity and understanding; otherwise our civilization will stagnate and die."

1. STATEMENT OF TERMS OF APPOINTMENT

(a) The terms and conditions of every appointment to the faculty will be stated or confirmed in writing, and a copy of the appointment document will be supplied to the faculty member. Any subsequent extensions or modifications of an appointment, and any special understandings, or any notices incumbent upon either party to provide, will be stated or confirmed in writing and a copy will be given to the faculty member.

(b) With the exception of special appointments clearly limited to a brief association with the institution, and reappointments of retired faculty members on special conditions, all full-time faculty appointments are of two kinds: (1) probationary appointments; (2) appointments with continuous tenure.

(c) Except for faculty members who have tenure status, every person with a teaching or research appointment of any kind will be informed each year in writing of the renewal of the appointment and of all matters relative to eligibility for the acquisition of tenure.

2. PROBATIONARY APPOINTMENTS

(a) Probationary appointments may be for one year, or for other stated periods, subject to renewal. The total period of full-time service prior to the acquisition of continuous tenure will not exceed _____ years,[1] including all previous full-time service with the rank of instructor or higher in other institutions of higher learning [*except* that the probationary period may extend to as much as four years, even if the total full-time service in the profession thereby exceeds seven years; the terms of such extension will be stated in writing at the time of initial appointment].[2] Scholarly leave of absence for one year or less will count as part of the probationary period as if it were prior service at another institution, unless the individual and the institution agree in writing to an exception to this provision at the time the leave is granted.

(b) The faculty member will be advised, at the time of initial appointment, of the substantive standards and procedures generally employed in decisions affecting renewal and tenure. Any special standards adopted by the faculty member's department or school will also be transmitted. The faculty member will be advised of the time when decisions affecting renewal or tenure are ordinarily made, and will be given the opportunity to submit material believed to be helpful to an adequate consideration of the faculty member's circumstances.

(c) Regardless of the stated term or other provisions of any appointments, written notice that a probationary appointment is not to be renewed will be given to the faculty member in advance of the expiration of the appointment, as follows: (1) not later than March 1 of the first academic year of service if the appointment expires at the end of that year; or, if a one-year appointment terminates during an academic year, at least three months in advance of its termination; (2) not later than December 15 of the second academic year of service if the appointment expires at the end of that year; or, if an initial two-year appointment terminates during an academic year, at least six months in advance of its termination; (3) at least twelve months before the expiration of an appointment after two or more years of service at the institution. The institution will normally notify faculty members of the terms and conditions of their renewals by March 15, but in no case will such information be given later than_____.[3]

(d) When a faculty recommendation or a decision not to renew an appointment has first been reached, the faculty member involved will be informed of that recommendation or decision in writing by the body or individual making the initial recommendation or decision; the faculty member will be advised upon request of the reasons which contributed to that decision. The faculty member may request a reconsideration by the recommending or deciding body.

(e) If the faculty member so requests, the reasons given in explanation of the nonrenewal will be confirmed in writing.

(f) Insofar as the faculty member alleges that the decision against renewal by the appropriate faculty body was based on inadequate consideration, the committee[4] which reviews the faculty member's allegation will determine whether the decision was the result of adequate consideration in terms of the relevant standards of the institution. The review committee will not substitute its judgment on the merits for that of the faculty body. If this committee, which can be the grievance committee noted in Regulation 15, is to be an elected faculty body. Similarly, the members of the committees noted in Regulations 4(c)(2), 4(d)(3), and 10 are to be elected. A committee of faculty members appointed by an appropriate elected faculty body can substitute for a committee that is elected directly. If the review committee believes that adequate consideration was not given to the faculty member's qualifications, it will request reconsideration by the faculty body, indicating the respects in which it believes the consideration may have been inadequate. It will provide copies of its findings to the faculty member, the faculty body, and the president or other appropriate administrative officer.

3. TERMINATION OF APPOINTMENT BY FACULTY MEMBERS

Faculty members may terminate their appointments effective at the end of an academic year, provided that they give notice in writing at the earliest possible opportunity, but not later than May 15, or thirty days after receiving notification of the terms of appointment for the coming year, whichever date occurs later. Faculty members may properly request a waiver of this requirement of notice in case of hardship or in a situation where they would otherwise be denied substantial professional advancement or other opportunity.

4. TERMINATION OF APPOINTMENTS BY THE INSTITUTION

(a) Termination of an appointment with continuous tenure, or of a probationary or special appointment before the end of the specified term, may be effected by the institution only for adequate cause.

(b) If termination takes the form of a dismissal for cause, it will be pursuant to the procedures specified in Regulation 5.

Financial Exigency

(c) (1) Termination of an appointment with continuous tenure, or of a probationary or special appointment before the end of the specified term, may occur under extraordinary circumstances because of a demonstrably bona fide financial exigency, i.e., an imminent financial crisis which threatens the survival of the institution as a whole and which cannot be alleviated by less drastic means.

[NOTE: Each institution in adopting regulations on financial exigency will need to decide how to share and allocate the hard judgments and decisions that are necessary in such a crisis.

As a first step, there should be a faculty body which participates in the decision that a condition of financial exigency exists or is imminent,[5] and that all feasible alternatives to termination of appointments have been pursued.

Judgments determining where within the overall academic program termination of appointments may occur involve considerations of educational policy, including affirmative action, as well as of faculty status, and should therefore be the primary responsibility of the faculty or of an appropriate faculty body.[6] The faculty or an appropriate faculty body should also exercise primary responsibility in determining the criteria for identifying the individuals whose appointments are to be terminated. These criteria may appropriately include considerations of length of service.

The responsibility for identifying individuals whose appointments are to be terminated should be committed to a person or group designated or approved by the faculty. The allocation of this responsibility may vary according to the size and character of the institution, the extent of the terminations to be made, or other considerations of fairness in judgment. The case of a faculty member given notice of proposed termination of appointment will be governed by the following procedure.]

140

(2) If the administration issues notice to a particular faculty member of an intention to terminate the appointment because of financial exigency, the faculty member will have the right to a full hearing before a faculty committee. The hearing need not conform in all respects with a proceeding conducted pursuant to Regulation 5, but the essentials of an on-the-record adjudicative hearing will be observed. The issues in this hearing may include:

(i) The existence and extent of the condition of financial exigency. The burden will rest on the administration to prove the existence and extent of the condition. The findings of a faculty committee in a previous proceeding involving the same issue may be introduced.

(ii) The validity of the educational judgments and the criteria for identification for termination; but the recommendations of a faculty body on these matters will be considered presumptively valid.

(iii) Whether the criteria are being properly applied in the individual case.

(3) If the institution, because of financial exigency, terminates appointments, it will not at the same time make new appointments except in extraordinary circumstances where a serious distortion in the academic program would otherwise result. The appointment of a faculty member with tenure will not be terminated in favor of retaining a faculty member without tenure, except in extraordinary circumstances where a serious distortion of the academic program would otherwise result.

(4) Before terminating an appointment because of financial exigency, the institution, with faculty participation, will make every effort to place the faculty member concerned in another suitable position within the institution.

(5) In all cases of termination of appointment because of financial exigency, the faculty member concerned will be given notice or severance salary not less than as prescribed in Regulation 8.

(6) In all cases of termination of appointment because of financial exigency, the place of the faculty member concerned will not be filled by a replacement within a period of three years,

unless the released faculty member has been offered reinstatement and a reasonable time in which to accept or decline it.

Discontinuance of Program or Department Not Mandated by Financial Exigency[7]

(d) Termination of an appointment with continuous tenure, or of a probationary or special appointment before the end of the specified term, may occur as a result of bona fide formal discontinuance of a program or department of instruction. The following standards and procedures will apply.

(1) The decision to discontinue formally a program or department of instruction will be based essentially upon educational considerations, as determined primarily by the faculty as a whole or an appropriate committee thereof.

[NOTE: "Educational considerations" do not include cyclical or temporary variations in enrollment. They must reflect long-range judgments that the educational mission of the institution as a whole will be enhanced by the discontinuance.]

(2) Before the administration issues notice to a faculty member of its intention to terminate an appointment because of formal discontinuance of a program or department of instruction, the institution will make every effort to place the faculty member concerned in another suitable position. If placement in another position would be facilitated by a reasonable period of training, financial and other support for such training will be proffered. If no position is available within the institution, with or without retraining, the faculty member's appointment then may be terminated, but only with provision for severance salary equitably adjusted to the faculty member's length of past and potential service.

[NOTE: When an institution proposes to discontinue a program or department of instruction, it should plan to bear the costs of relocating, training, or otherwise compensating faculty members adversely affected.]

(3) A faculty member may appeal a proposed relocation or termination resulting from a discontinuance and has a right to a full hearing before a faculty committee. The hearing need not conform in all respects with a proceeding conducted pursuant to Regulation 5, but the essentials of an on-the-record adjudicative

hearing will be observed. The issues in such a hearing may include the institution's failure to satisfy any of the conditions specified in Regulation 4(d). In such a hearing a faculty determination that a program or department is to be discontinued will be considered presumptively valid, but the burden of proof on other issues will rest on the administration.

Termination Because of Physical or Mental Disability

(e) Termination of an appointment with tenure, or of a probationary or special appointment before the end of the period of appointment, because of physical or mental disability, will be based upon clear and convincing medical evidence that the faculty member, even with reasonable accommodation, is no longer able to perform the essential duties of the position. The decision to terminate will be reached only after there has been appropriate consultation and after the faculty member concerned, or someone representing the faculty member, has been informed of the basis of the proposed action and has been afforded an opportunity to present the faculty member's position and to respond to the evidence. If the faculty member so requests, the evidence will be reviewed by the Faculty Committee on Academic Freedom and Tenure [or whatever title it may have] before a final decision is made by the governing board on the recommendation of the administration. The faculty member will be given severance salary not less than as prescribed in Regulation 8.

Review

(f) In cases of termination of appointment, the governing board will be available for ultimate review.

5. DISMISSAL PROCEDURES

(a) Adequate cause for a dismissal will be related, directly and substantially, to the fitness of faculty members in their professional capacities as teachers or researchers. Dismissal will not be used to restrain faculty members in their exercise of academic freedom or other rights of American citizens.

(b) Dismissal of a faculty member with continuous tenure, or with a special or probationary appointment before the end of the specified term, will be preceded by: (1) discussions between the faculty member and appropriate administrative officers looking toward a mutual settlement; (2) informal inquiry by the duly elected faculty committee [insert name of committee] which may, failing to effect an adjustment, determine whether in its opinion dismissal proceedings should be undertaken, without its opinion being binding upon the president; (3) a statement of charges, framed with reasonable particularity by the president or the president's delegate.

(c) A dismissal, as defined in Regulation 5(a), will be preceded by a statement of reasons, and the individual concerned will have the right to be heard initially by the elected faculty hearing committee [insert name of committee].[8] Members deeming themselves disqualified for bias or interest will remove themselves from the case, either at the request of a party or on their own initiative. Each party will have a maximum of two challenges without stated cause.[9]

(1) Pending a final decision by the hearing committee, the faculty member will be suspended, or assigned to other duties in lieu of suspension, only if immediate harm to the faculty member or others is threatened by continuance. Before suspending a faculty member, pending an ultimate determination of the faculty member's status through the institution's hearing procedures, the administration will consult with the Faculty Committee on Academic Freedom and Tenure [or whatever other title it may have] concerning the propriety, the length, and the other conditions of the suspension. A suspension which is intended to be final is a dismissal, and will be treated as such. Salary will continue during the period of the suspension.

(2) The hearing committee may, with the consent of the parties concerned, hold joint prehearing meetings with the parties in order to (i) simplify the issues, (ii) effect stipulations of facts, (iii) provide for the exchange of documentary or other information, and (iv) achieve such other appropriate prehearing objectives as will make the hearing fair, effective, and expeditious.

(3) Service of notice of hearing with specific charges in writing will be made at least twenty days prior to the hearing. The faculty member may waive a hearing or may respond to the charges in writing at any time before the hearing. If the faculty

member waives a hearing, but denies the charges or asserts that the charges do not support a finding of adequate cause, the hearing tribunal will evaluate all available evidence and rest its recommendation upon the evidence in the record.

(4) The committee, in consultation with the president and the faculty member, will exercise its judgment as to whether the hearing should be public or private.

(5) During the proceedings the faculty member will be permitted to have an academic advisor and counsel of the faculty member's choice.

(6) At the request of either party or the hearing committee, a representative of a responsible educational association will be permitted to attend the proceedings as an observer.

(7) A verbatim record of the hearing or hearings will be taken and a typewritten copy will be made available to the faculty member without cost, at the faculty member's request.

(8) The burden of proof that adequate cause exists rests with the institution and will be satisfied only by clear and convincing evidence in the record considered as a whole.

(9) The hearing committee will grant adjournments to enable either party to investigate evidence as to which a valid claim of surprise is made.

(10) The faculty member will be afforded an opportunity to obtain necessary witnesses and documentary or other evidence. The administration will cooperate with the hearing committee in securing witnesses and making available documentary and other evidence.

(11) The faculty member and the administration will have the right to confront and cross-examine all witnesses. Where the witnesses cannot or will not appear, but the committee determines that the interests of justice require admission of their statements, the committee will identify the witnesses, disclose their statements, and, if possible, provide for interrogatories.

(12) In the hearing of charges of incompetence, the testimony will include that of qualified faculty members from this or other institutions of higher education.

(13) The hearing committee will not be bound by strict rules of legal evidence, and may admit any evidence which is of

probative value in determining the issues involved. Every possible effort will be made to obtain the most reliable evidence available.

(14) The findings of fact and the decision will be based solely on the hearing record.

(15) Except for such simple announcements as may be required, covering the time of the hearing and similar matters, public statements and publicity about the case by either the faculty member or administrative officers will be avoided so far as possible until the proceedings have been completed, including consideration by the governing board of the institution. The president and the faculty member will be notified of the decision in writing and will be given a copy of the record of the hearing.

(16) If the hearing committee concludes that adequate cause for dismissal has not been established by the evidence in the record, it will so report to the president. If the president rejects the report, the president will state the reasons for doing so, in writing, to the hearing committee and to the faculty member, and provide an opportunity for response before transmitting the case to the governing board. If the hearing committee concludes that adequate cause for a dismissal has been established, but that an academic penalty less than dismissal would be more appropriate, it will so recommend, with supporting reasons.

6. ACTION BY THE GOVERNING BOARD

If dismissal or other severe sanction is recommended, the president will, on request of the faculty member, transmit to the governing board the record of the case. The governing board's review will be based on the record of the committee hearing, and it will provide opportunity for argument, oral or written or both, by the principals at the hearings or by their representatives. The decision of the hearing committee will either be sustained or the proceeding returned to the committee with specific objections. The committee will then reconsider, taking into account the stated objections and receiving new evidence if necessary. The governing board will make a final decision only after study of the committee's reconsideration.

7. PROCEDURES FOR IMPOSITION OF SANCTIONS OTHER THAN DISMISSAL

(a) If the administration believes that the conduct of a faculty member, although not constituting adequate cause for dismissal, is sufficiently grave to justify imposition of a severe sanction, such as suspension from service for a stated period, the administration may institute a proceeding to impose such a severe sanction; the procedures outlined in Regulation 5 will govern such a proceeding.

(b) If the administration believes that the conduct of a faculty member justifies imposition of a minor sanction, such as a reprimand, it will notify the faculty member of the basis of the proposed sanction and provide the faculty member with an opportunity to persuade the administration that the proposed sanction should not be imposed. A faculty member who believes that a major sanction has been incorrectly imposed under this paragraph, or that a minor sanction has been unjustly imposed, may, pursuant to Regulation 15, petition the faculty grievance committee for such action as may be appropriate.

8. TERMINAL SALARY OR NOTICE

If the appointment is terminated, the faculty member will receive salary or notice in accordance with the following schedule: at least three months, if the final decision is reached by March 1 (or three months prior to the expiration) of the first year of probationary service; at least six months, if the decision is reached by December 15 of the second year (or after nine months but prior to eighteen months) of probationary service; at least one year, if the decision is reached after eighteen months of probationary service or if the faculty member has tenure. This provision for terminal notice or salary need not apply in the event that there has been a finding that the conduct which justified dismissal involved moral turpitude. On the recommendation of the faculty hearing committee or the president, the governing board, in determining what, if any, payments will be made beyond the effective date of dismissal, may take into account the length and quality of service of the faculty member.

9. ACADEMIC FREEDOM AND PROTECTION AGAINST DISCRIMINATION

(a) All members of the faculty, whether tenured or not, are entitled to academic freedom as set forth in the 1940 *Statement of Principles on Academic Freedom and Tenure,* formulated by the Association of American Colleges and the American Association of University Professors.

(b) All members of the faculty, whether tenured or not, are entitled to protection against illegal or unconstitutional discrimination by the institution, or discrimination on a basis not demonstrably related to the faculty member's professional performance, including but not limited to race, sex, religion, national origin, age, disability, marital status, or sexual orientation.

10. COMPLAINTS OF VIOLATION OF ACADEMIC FREEDOM OR OF DISCRIMINATION IN NONREAPPOINTMENT

If a faculty member on probationary or other nontenured appointment alleges that a decision against reappointment was based significantly on considerations violative of (a) academic freedom or (b) governing policies on making appointments without prejudice with respect to race, sex, religion, national origin, age, disability, marital status, or sexual orientation, the allegation will be given preliminary consideration by the [insert name of committee], which will seek to settle the matter by informal methods. The allegation will be accompanied by a statement that the faculty member agrees to the presentation, for the consideration of the faculty committees, of such reasons and evidence as the institution may allege in support of its decision. If the difficulty is unresolved at this stage, and if the committee so recommends, the matter will be heard in the manner set forth in Regulations 5 and 6, except that the faculty member making the complaint is responsible for stating the grounds upon which the allegations are based, and the burden of proof will rest upon the faculty member. If the faculty member succeeds in establishing a prima facie case, it is incumbent upon those who made the decision against reappointment to come forward with evidence in support of their decision. Statistical evidence of improper discrimination may be used in establishing a prima facie case.

11. ADMINISTRATIVE PERSONNEL

The foregoing regulations apply to administrative personnel who hold academic rank, but only in their capacity as faculty members. Administrators who allege that a consideration violative of academic freedom, or of governing policies against improper discrimination as stated in Regulation 10, significantly contributed to a decision to terminate their appointment to an administrative post, or not to reappoint them, are entitled to the procedures set forth in Regulation 10.

12. POLITICAL ACTIVITIES OF FACULTY MEMBERS

Faculty members, as citizens, are free to engage in political activities. Where necessary, leaves of absence may be given for the duration of an election campaign or a term of office, on timely application, and for a reasonable period of time. The terms of such leave of absence will be set forth in writing, and the leave will not affect unfavorably the tenure status of a faculty member, except that time spent on such leave will not count as probationary service unless otherwise agreed to.[10]

[NOTE: Regulations 13, 14, and 15 are suggested in tentative form, and will require adaptation to the specific structure and operations of the institution; the provisions as recommended here are intended only to indicate the nature of the provisions to be included, and not to offer specific detail.]

13. GRADUATE STUDENT ACADEMIC STAFF

(a) The terms and conditions of every appointment to a graduate or teaching assistantship will be stated in writing, and a copy of the appointment document will be supplied to the graduate or teaching assistant.

(b) In no case will a graduate or teaching assistant be dismissed without having been provided with a statement of reasons and an opportunity to be heard before a duly constituted committee. (A dismissal is a termination before the end of the period of appointment.)

(c) A graduate or teaching assistant who establishes a prima facie case to the satisfaction of a duly constituted committee that a decision against reappointment was based significantly on considerations violative of academic freedom, or of governing policies against improper discrimination as stated in Regulation 10, will be given a statement of reasons by those responsible for the nonreappointment and an opportunity to be heard by the committee.

(d) Graduate or teaching assistants will have access to the faculty grievance committee, as provided in Regulation 15.

14. OTHER ACADEMIC STAFF

(a) In no case will a member of the academic staff[11] who is not otherwise protected by the preceding regulations which relate to dismissal proceedings be dismissed without having been provided with a statement of reasons and an opportunity to be heard before a duly constituted committee. (A dismissal is a termination before the end of the period of appointment.)

(b) With respect to the nonreappointment of a member of such academic staff who establishes a prima facie case to the satisfaction of a duly constituted committee that a consideration violative of academic freedom, or of governing policies against improper discrimination as stated in Regulation 10, significantly contributed to the nonreappointment, the academic staff member will be given a statement of reasons by those responsible for the nonreappointment and an opportunity to be heard by the committee.

15. GRIEVANCE PROCEDURE

If any faculty member alleges cause for grievance in any matter not covered by the procedures described in the foregoing regulations, the faculty member may petition the elected faculty grievance committee [here name the committee] for redress. The petition will set forth in detail the nature of the grievance and will state against whom the grievance is directed. It will contain any factual or other data which the petitioner deems pertinent to the case. Statistical evidence of improper discrimination, including discrimination in salary, may be used in establishing a prima facie case. The committee will decide whether or not the facts merit a detailed investigation; if the faculty member succeeds in establishing a prima facie case, it is incumbent upon those who made the decision to come forward with evidence in support of their decision. Submission of a petition will not automatically entail investigation or detailed consideration thereof. The committee may seek to bring about a settlement of the issue(s) satisfactory to the parties. If in the opinion of the committee such a settlement is not possible or is not appropriate, the committee will report its findings and recommendations to the petitioner and to the appropriate administrative officer and faculty body, and the petitioner will, upon request, be provided an opportunity to present the grievance to them. The grievance committee will consist of three [or some other number] elected members of the faculty. No officer of administration will serve on the committee.

NOTE ON IMPLEMENTATION

The *Recommended Institutional Regulations* here presented will require for their implementation a number of structural arrangements and agencies. For example, the *Regulations* will need support by:

(a) channels of communication among all the involved components of the institution, and between them and a concerned faculty member;

(b) definitions of corporate and individual faculty status within the college or university government, and of the role of the faculty in decisions relating to academic freedom and tenure; and

(c) appropriate procedures for the creation and operation of faculty committees, with particular regard to the principles of faculty authority and responsibility.

The forms which these supporting elements assume will of course vary from one institution to another. Consequently, no detailed description of the elements is attempted in these *Recommended Institutional Regulations.* With respect to the principles involved, guidance will be found in the Association's 1966 *Statement on Government of Colleges and Universities.*

Endnotes:
1. Under the "1940 Statement of Principles on Academic Freedom and Tenure," this period may not exceed seven years.
2. The exception here noted applies only to an institution whose maximum probationary period exceeds four years.

3. April 15 is the recommended date.
4. This committee, which can be the grievance committee noted in Regulation 15, is to be an elected faculty body. Similarly, the members of the committees noted in Regulations 4(c)(2), 4(d)(3), and 10 are to be elected. A committee of faculty members appointed by an appropriate elected faculty body can substitute for a committee that is elected directly.
5. See "The Role of the Faculty in Budgetary and Salary Matters" (AAUP, *Policy Documents and Reports,* 9th ed. [Washington, D.C., 2001], 232–35), especially the following passages:

> The faculty should participate both in the preparation of the total institutional budget and (within the framework of the total budget) in decisions relevant to the further apportioning of its specific fiscal divisions (salaries, academic programs, tuition, physical plant and grounds, etc.). The soundness of resulting decisions should be enhanced if an elected representative committee of the faculty participates in deciding on the overall allocation of institutional resources and the proportion to be devoted directly to the academic program. This committee should be given access to all information that it requires to perform its task effectively, and it should have the opportunity to confer periodically with representatives of the administration and governing board. . . .

> Circumstances of financial exigency obviously pose special problems. At institutions experiencing major threats to their continued financial support, the faculty should be informed as early and specifically as possible of significant impending financial difficulties. The faculty—with substantial representation from its nontenured as well as its tenured members, since it is the former who are likely to bear the brunt of the reduction—should participate at the department, college or professional school, and institution-wide levels in key decisions as to the future of the institution and of specific academic programs within the institution. The faculty, employing accepted standards of due process, should

assume primary responsibility for determining the status of individual faculty members.

6. See "Statement on Government of Colleges and Universities" (*Policy Documents and Reports,* 217–23), especially the following passage:

    Faculty status and related matters are primarily a faculty responsibility; this area includes appointments, reappointments, decisions not to reappoint, promotions, the granting of tenure, and dismissal. The primary responsibility of the faculty for such matters is based upon the fact that its judgment is central to general educational policy.

7. When discontinuance of a program or department is mandated by financial exigency of the institution, the standards of Regulation 4(c) above will apply.

8. This committee should not be the same as the committee referred to in Regulation 5(b)(2).

9. Regulations of the institution should provide for alternates, or for some other method of filling vacancies on the hearing committee resulting from disqualification, challenge without stated cause, illness, resignation, or other reason.

10. See "Statement on Professors and Political Activity," *Policy Documents and Reports,* 33–34.

11. Each institution should define with particularity who are members of the academic staff.

AAUP Recommended Institutional Regulations on Academic Freedom and Tenure are available from http://www.aaup.org/statements/Redbook/Rbrir.htm

Nursing Faculty Shortage Information

White Paper

May 2003

Faculty Shortages in Baccalaureate and Graduate Nursing Programs: Scope of the Problem and Strategies for Expanding the Supply

The American Association of Colleges of Nursing (AACN) recognizes that the shortage of faculty in schools of nursing with baccalaureate and graduate programs is a continuing and expanding problem. Over the past several years, the deficit of faculty has reached critical proportions as the current faculty workforce rapidly advances toward retirement and the pool of younger replacement faculty decreases. The purpose of this white paper is to summarize the scope of the problem, discuss issues contributing to the shortage of faculty, and put forth strategies for expanding the capacity of the current and future pool of nursing faculty.

Section I. Scope and Significance of the Problem

The United States is in the midst of an unprecedented shortage of registered nurses. This shortage is expected to persist because of the increasing demand for health care as baby boomers approach retirement; the aging nursing workforce; and the decline of interest in nursing as a career because of expanding opportunities for women in previously male-dominant professions (Staiger, Auerbach, & Buerhaus, 2000).

According to projections from the Bureau of Labor Statistics (BLS), there will be more than one million vacant positions for registered nurses (RNs) by 2010 due to growth in demand for nursing care and net replacements due to retirement (Hecker, 2001). Data from the 2000 National Sample Survey of Registered Nurses estimated that 39 percent of RNs employed in nursing held baccalaureate or master's degrees in nursing (Spratley, Johnson, Sochalski, *et al.,* 2001). Therefore, one can postulate that *at least* 390,000 of the vacancies projected by the BLS will be for RNs with baccalaureate or master's nursing degrees, which translates into the need for large numbers of well-prepared faculty to educate these new nurses. In addition, US high schools will graduate the largest class in history in 2007-2008—a projected 3.2 million graduates (Western Interstate Commission for Higher Education, 1998). Even if enrollment demand in nursing increases only modestly, will sufficient numbers of nursing faculty be available to teach these students?

Intensifying the overall nursing shortage is the increasing deficit of full-time master's and doctorally prepared nursing faculty. Unfortunately, even now the shortage of faculty is contributing to the current nursing shortage by limiting the number of students admitted to nursing programs. In 2002, an AACN survey determined that 5,283 qualified applications to baccalaureate, master's, and doctoral programs were not accepted; and an insufficient number of faculty was cited by 41.7 percent of responding schools as a reason for not accepting all qualified applicants (Berlin, Stennett, & Bednash, 2003a). A special survey was conducted by AACN in 2000 to determine the vacancy rate for faculty. In a national sample of 220 schools (38% of AACN-member institutions), there were 5,132 full-time faculty positions. Of these positions, 379 (7.4%) were vacant. The mean number of vacancies per school was 1.7 with a range of 0-17, while only 20 schools reported no vacancies (AACN, 2000). Other studies corroborate these findings. A Texas study found a vacancy rate of 4.7 percent for full-time equivalent (FTE) faculty positions in baccalaureate and advanced practice programs (29 of 617 positions); and a California study identified the need for 163 FTE faculty or 9.2 percent of the total statewide baccalaureate and higher degree program faculty by 2003 (Furino, Gott, & Miller, 2000; California Strategic Planning Committee for Nursing, 2001). In addition, a southeast regional study found vacancy

155

rates of 5.7% for associate degree, baccalaureate, and graduate programs at the beginning of the 2000-2001 school year (Council on Collegiate Education for Nursing, 2002). To the casual observer, vacancy rates of less than 10 percent may not seem significant, but even one or two vacant positions in a school can have a considerable impact on the didactic and clinical teaching workload of the remaining faculty.

Section II. Factors Contributing to the Shortage of Faculty

A. Faculty Age

Although there are multiple factors contributing to the shortage of faculty, the impact of faculty age and retirement timelines coupled with an inadequate pool of younger faculty for replacement are the primary influences on future faculty availability. AACN conducts a survey of faculty in baccalaureate and higher degree granting schools of nursing each fall. In 2002, surveys were sent to 682 schools. There were 9,978 full-time nurse faculty in 555 (81.4%) responding institutions. The proportion of doctoral and master's prepared faculty was 49.9 and 50.1 percent, respectively. Of those with doctoral degrees, 59.5 percent held doctorates in

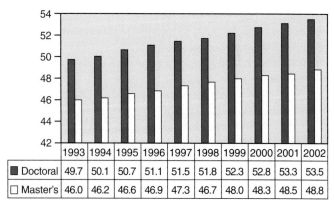

	1993	1994	1995	1996	1997	1998	1999	2000	2001	2002
■ Doctoral	49.7	50.1	50.7	51.1	51.5	51.8	52.3	52.8	53.3	53.5
□ Master's	46.0	46.2	46.6	46.9	47.3	46.7	48.0	48.3	48.5	48.8

Figure 1. Mean age of full-time nurse faculty, 1993-2002. Age data not collected in 1996; midpoint of '95 and '97 used. Source: American Association of Colleges of Nursing, 1993-2002 (c) 2003.

nursing, whereas 40.5 percent had degrees in other fields (Berlin, Stennett, & Bednash, 2003b). Like the overall nursing workforce, mean age has increased steadily, from 49.7 years in 1993 to 53.3 in 2002 for doctoral faculty and 46 to 48.8 for master's faculty.

1. Faculty Retirement Projections. Regression analysis of faculty 62 years and younger found that the mean age was increasing at almost half a year per year (0.43) for full-time doctorally prepared faculty. Retirement projections for individuals who were faculty in 2001 revealed that from 2004 through 2012, between 200 and 300 doctorally prepared faculty will be eligible for retirement annually. The modal year of retirement is 2009 (Berlin & Sechrist, 2002a). The mean age for the 2001 full-time master's faculty cohort was increasing a third of a year per year (0.33), and from 2012 through 2018 between 220 and 280 master's faculty will be eligible to retire each year; the modal retirement year is 2015 (Berlin & Sechrist, 2002b). These projections represent the best case scenario, based on the conservative assumptions that faculty will work until age 62 and that there will be no additional departures from academic life.

2. Faculty Age Groups. In conjunction with the increase in mean age, the proportion of full-time doctorally prepared

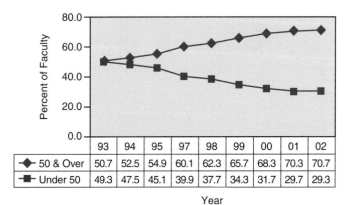

Year	93	94	95	97	98	99	00	01	02
50 & Over	50.7	52.5	54.9	60.1	62.3	65.7	68.3	70.3	70.7
Under 50	49.3	47.5	45.1	39.9	37.7	34.3	31.7	29.7	29.3

Year

Figure 2. Percent of full-time doctorally prepared faculty over and under the age of 50 for each reporting year. Source: Berlin & Sechrist, 2002a; Berlin & Sechrist, 2003b.

faculty age 50 and over and under 50 has changed dramatically. In 1993, the proportion of faculty under and over age 50 was almost equal; in 2002 the percentage of those 50 and over increased by 20 percent (Berlin & Sechrist, 2002a; Berlin & Sechrist, 2003a). Full-time master's faculty 50 and over increased from 32.6 to 46.9 percent during the same time period.

B. Departure from Academic Life

1. Decline in Percent of Younger Faculty. From 1993–2002, the percentage of doctorally prepared faculty members in the age categories of 46–55, 56–65, and over 65 years increased by 2.6 percent, 14.5 percent, and 1.6 percent, respectively. In contrast, there were decreases in the age groups 35 years and younger (0.6%) and 36–45 years (18.1%) (Fig. 3). The decline in the 36–45 year group of doctorally prepared faculty is particularly trouble-some, given that "the doctoral degree should be considered the appropriate and desired credential for a career as a nurse educa-tor" (AACN, 1996, p. 3). Advancement to the next age category accounts for some of the decline, but egression from academic life is the major reason for the loss of younger faculty members. Master's prepared faculty in the 36-45 year group showed the same pattern of decline (Berlin & Sechrist, 2003d).

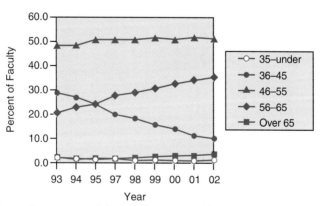

Figure 3. Percent of doctorally prepared full-time faculty in each age category, 1993–2002. Source: Berlin & Sechrist, 2002a; Berlin & Sechrist, 2003c.

In the 280 schools reporting faculty resignation and retirement data in 2002, 188 full-time doctorally prepared faculty and 202 master's prepared faculty resigned from schools of nursing. Nineteen individuals with doctoral preparation and 62 with master's preparation were between the ages of 36 and 45 years of age. Of those, subsequent employment plans were reported for 16 doctoral and 58 master's resignees. Although over one-half (56.2%) of those with doctoral degrees left to take other school of nursing faculty or administrative positions, seven individuals (43.8%) left academia to assume non-academic positions such as nursing service, private sector, or private practice positions. Forty-three percent (25 individuals) of those with master's preparation resigned to take non-academic jobs (AACN, 2002b).

2. Employment of Doctoral Graduates. Of the 457 doctoral graduates in 2001-2002, almost 27 percent (28.6%) reported employment commitments in settings other than schools of nursing (Berlin, Stennett, & Bednash, 2003a). This finding is confirmed by data from two additional sources. Data from the Survey of Earned Doctorates indicated that the percent of nursing doctoral recipients planning to be employed in areas other than education increased steadily from 15.5 percent in the time period 1980 through 1984 to 26.9 percent from 1995-1999. Further, teaching as a primary employment activity decreased from 70.8 percent to 59.5 percent during the same two time periods (National Opinion Research Center, 2001). The National Sample Survey of Registered Nurses databases estimated that in 1992, 1996, and 2000 the proportion of nurses with nursing doctorates who were employed in schools of nursing with baccalaureate and higher degrees showed steady declines, going from 68 percent in 1992 to 49 percent in 2000 (Division of Nursing, 2001).

C. Salary Differentials

Salary is an influential factor in the employment decisions of those completing graduate education. In a comparison of responsibilities and salaries associated with various employment opportunities, faculty positions may not be as appealing as other offers. Average salaries for clinical positions have risen more than those for faculty positions because most universities are constrained in their ability to increase faculty salaries (Brendtro & Hegge, 2000; AACN, 1999a). Academic institutions, especially those faced with budget cuts, generally cannot compete with nonacademic employers. In fall 2002, the median academic-year salaries for instructional faculty with doctoral degrees with the ranks of associate and assistant professors were $61,000 and $53,355 respectively; for those with master's degrees the median salaries were $49,546 and $45,214 (Berlin, Stennett, & Bednash, 2003b). A sample of clinical and administrative nursing salaries is presented in Table 1 (Salary.Com, 2003). Since the clinical and administrative salaries are based on a calendar year, academic salaries were converted to a calendar year basis. (Academic salaries are multiplied by 11/9 or 1.22 to convert to calendar year salaries.)

Salary may also be a determinant in the decision of master's prepared nurses to return to doctoral study. Potential students calculate whether it profits them to seek doctoral study and enter academia when they can earn better salaries in non-academic master's-level positions.

Tuition and Loan Burden for Graduate Study

Average tuition, required fees, room/board, and percent of loan burden for graduate students by type of institution are presented in Table 2 (Peterson's Colleges of Nursing Database, 2002). In addition to the basic student charges, additional costs include textbooks, medical equipment, uniforms or laboratory coats, transportation to/from clinical sites, and thesis and dissertation expenses. Also, net income foregone is a consideration as the amount may be substantial, especially for full-time study.

E. Diminishing Pipeline of Enrollees and Graduates

Five-year trend data in a cohort of 76 schools reporting data each year to AACN from 1998-2002 showed an average increase of 31 doctoral students per year ($P = 0.005$). The pattern of graduations, however, indicated no trend (Berlin, Stennett, & Bednash, 2003a).

Table 1. Comparison of full-time, calendar year instructional nurse faculty salaries and selected non-academic base salaries, 2002–2003, all US

School of Nursing

Instructional Faculty Positions:	Median	75th Percentile
Associate Professor (Doctoral)	$74,556	$81,116
Associate Professor (Master's)	$60,556	$67,259
Assistant Professor (Doctoral)	$65,212	$69,795
Assistant Professor (Master's)	$55,262	$61,310

Administrative Faculty Positions:
Director* of baccalaureate or master's program

Associate Professor (Doctoral)	$78,852	$85,906
Associate Professor (Master's)	$64,163	$73,887
Assistant Professor (Doctoral)	$71,313	$77,081
Assistant Professor (Master's)	$67,472	$78,075

Dean** of nursing program

(Doctoral)	$90,000	$116,000
(Master's)	$63,528	$80,000

Clinical/Administrative Positions:

Chief Nurse Anesthetist	$128,879	$139,625
VP for Nursing	$113,100	$134,122
Nurse Anesthetist	$105,890	$114,647
Nursing Director	$93,344	$103,083
NPs (Specialty Care)	$69,407	$76,407
Nurse Manager	$69,416	$75,326
Head Nurse (Critical Care)	$68,194	$75,105
Clinical Nurse Specialist	$61,351	$69,666

Sources: Berlin, L.E., Stennett, J., & Bednash, G.D. (2002a); Salary.Com (March 2002); and Tumolo J. & Collins, A. (2001).

*The term director refers to an administrative faculty member who is responsible for a program within the school of nursing, not the dean.

**The term dean refers to the chief executive officer of a school of nursing and encompasses titles such as director, chair, head, and coordinator.

Table 2. Average tuition, required fees, room and board, and percent of students receiving financial aid: graduate students by type of institution, academic year 2001-2002.*

Public Institutions	Average
Tuition (In-State Resident)	$3,659
Required Fees	$769
Room and Board (on campus)	$5,009
Percent of Students with Financial Aid	49.2%

Private Institutions	Average
Tuition	$11,020
Required Fees	$441
Room and Board (on campus)	$6,799
Percent of Students with Financial Aid	56.4%

*Peterson's Colleges of Nursing Database, 2002. Peterson's, a part of The Thomson Corporation. All rights reserved.

In the fall of 2002, there were 81 research-focused doctoral programs in nursing, with a total of 3,168 enrollees and 457 graduates. Fifty-five percent of enrollees were part-time students, the major reason that graduates represent only 12.8 percent of enrollees (Berlin, Stennett, & Bednash, 2003a). The failure of schools to produce more graduates is particularly disconcerting given that the number of doctoral programs has increased from 54 in 1992 to 83 (includes two clinically-focused programs) in 2002 (Berlin, Bednash, & Alsheimer, 1993; Berlin, Stennett, & Bednash, 2003a).

When evaluating the pipeline for doctoral preparation, trends in master's education must also be considered. In a five-year cohort of 289 schools reporting data each year, enrollments declined steadily from 1998-2001 followed by an increase of 898 students in 2002. Despite the increase this year, regression analysis indicated an average decrease of 110 students per year. Graduation patterns showed a steady decline of 249 graduates per year (P = 0.002). Graduations will continue to decline each year until the 2002 enrollees graduate (Berlin, Stennett, & Bednash, 2003a). This is noteworthy because master's graduates are the source of a significant percentage of current and future faculty, as well as the source for future doctoral students. It will be several years before the increase in master's enrollees is translated into increased graduates. However, the shift of master's prepared faculty to doctoral student status may not increase the number of new people in the faculty pool because many already are functioning in faculty roles.

F. Age of Doctoral Recipients and Time to Degree

Of the 365 recipients of nursing doctoral degrees in 1999 who reported age, the median age was 46.2 years. Almost half of all graduates (48.8%) were between the ages of 45 and 54 years; 12 percent were older than 55 years, and only 25 (6.8%) were under 35. In comparison, the median age of all research doctoral awardees in the US in 1999 was 33.7 years (National Opinion Research Center, 2001). Given that the mean age of retirement for full-time faculty in 2002 was 61.5 years, the number of productive teaching and research years are curtailed because of advanced age at graduation (AACN, 2002b). From 1999–2000, the mean number of years registered in a doctoral program was 8.3 years for nursing graduates compared to 6.8 years for all research awardees. Median time elapsed between entry in a master's program to completion of the doctorate in nursing was almost twice that of other fields, 15.9 and 8.5 years, respectively (National Opinion Research Center, 2001).

G. Faculty Workload and Role Expectation Issues

1. Job Dissatisfaction. The literature frequently cites dissatisfaction with workplace as a reason for the loss of younger faculty from academia (Brendtro & Hegge, 2000; DeYoung & Bliss, 1995; Ketefian, 1991). Initiatives aimed at increasing the number of faculty will not succeed if faculty are not satisfied and retained. In order to quantify the extent of job dissatisfaction, job satisfaction variables from the 1999 *National Study of Postsecondary*

Faculty (US Department of Education, 2001) were analyzed. Of the 1,073,667 postsecondary faculty in the database, there were an estimated 4,295 full-time nurse faculty holding doctoral degrees whose primary responsibilities consisted of teaching and research. The variables of interest were overall job satisfaction, job security, opportunity for advancement, workload, effectiveness of leadership, salary, benefits, and time to keep current in one's field. Percent of dissatisfaction was compared between two groups: (1) individuals holding the rank of full and associate professor and (2) individuals within the ranks of assistant, instructor, and lecturer. (The public use database would not allow further discrimination of ranks.) Findings revealed that junior faculty (assistant, instructor, and lecturer) reported higher percentages of dissatisfaction than did senior faculty on all variables except one. Junior faculty were not as dissatisfied as senior faculty regarding time available to keep current in one's field. The response to workload was most noteworthy. Dissatisfaction with workload was an estimated 54.7 percent for junior faculty, almost twice that of senior faculty (29.5%) (Berlin & Sechrist, 2003e).

 2. Role Expectations. Like all academic disciplines, changing faculty workload demands and role expectations are contributing to the nursing faculty shortage. Change is ever present: in the way higher education is conducted; in the traditional roles of teaching, scholarship, and service; and in the characteristics of today's students. These changes challenge faculty, require more time and preparation to be successful in the faculty role, and may cause those not sufficiently prepared to be dissatisfied and leave. The life of the college professor has changed considerably since the late 1980s (Longin, 2002). Describing the professoriate in transition, Berberet and McMillin (2002) highlight the varied responsibilities and stressors of faculty. In addition to the traditional teaching role, they assert that faculty also are expected to obtain extramural funding, conduct research, produce scholarship, and offer community and university service. Most full-time faculty spend extended hours advising and mentoring students outside the classroom, updating curricula, developing new courses, reading to remain current, and mastering new

164

advances in technology. With these multiple demands upon all faculty, "time is becoming their most precious commodity" (p. 2). In fact, in a recent survey, "73 percent of faculty respondents expressed frustration at 'never having time to complete a piece of work'" (p. 9).

3. Today's Student Population. Nontraditional students. In past years, the "traditional" nursing student was an eighteen year old high school graduate entering college directly from high school. Since 1995, the average age of graduates from all nursing programs is 30.9 years, an increase of seven years in the previous decade (Spratley, Johnson, Sochalski, *et al.,* 2001). Now, almost 73 percent of undergraduate students are considered "nontraditional" by virtue of their older age, more independent financial status, delayed entry into higher education, and competing responsibilities such as jobs and families. While the majority of students with the most nontraditional characteristics attend community colleges or private for-profit institutions, 14.4 and 19.0 percent attend public four-year and private not-for-profit institutions, respectively. Most students continue to pursue undergraduate education on a full-time basis, but the number of part-time students has tripled since 1970 (US Department of Education, 2002). Experienced faculty know that these more mature students commit a significant amount of time and energy to their work and family responsibilities. They demand a relevant, no-nonsense approach to education that is immediately applicable and complementary to their lives. Many mature students are gifted in their scholarship, motivation, life experiences, and insights. These characteristics often challenge faculty to plan more creative, practical, and interactive teaching-learning strategies such as case studies, problem-solving exercises, research projects, and service learning experiences. While these approaches may better meet the needs of mature students, they are time-intensive for faculty to develop and monitor.

Multi-generations. According to information gleaned from those who study the various generations, disconnects often occur between the values and characteristics of current older faculty and younger students, according to the age of each. For example, mature faculty members as a whole have very different views about work, authority, relationships, responsibility, and the nature of learning than today's twenty-something learners. These characteristic differences require new approaches to teaching—learning to meet the needs of various groups (Brown, 2001; Zemke, 2001).

Student capabilities. Faculty are challenged by the broad range of student capabilities in today's classrooms, ranging from at-risk to exceptional. Levine and Cureton (1998) describe the current generation of undergraduates, in general, as committed to doing well, but often lacking in basic skills necessary for college-level work. This observation is echoed anecdotally by numerous nursing academics. Even more serious, about one-third of high school students considered at risk for low academic attainment enroll in a four-year college within two years of high school graduation, despite their at-risk status (US Department of Education, 2002). Some of these students may wish to enroll in nursing programs. In order to be successful, students lacking in prerequisite skills often need additional academic help and other types of support. Remedial work for these students, while necessary, consumes valuable faculty time. At the other extreme, exceptional students may be eager for advanced or enrichment opportunities in their studies. Faculty generally are eager to help meet the needs of all students, but developing and implementing activities appropriate for different learner subgroups takes time and energy.

Study habits. Conventional wisdom and many school handbooks suggest three hours of student out-of-class preparation for every credit hour of class. This would be roughly 45 hours of study for 15 class hours per week (five courses of three hours each). However, Young (2002) reported a recent study that described the study habits of recent freshman classes at four-year residential colleges. Sixty three percent of full-time students reported studying 15 hours a week or less, and 19 percent spent only 1-5 hours per week studying. Mature faculty may expect students to demonstrate the self-directed study habits prevalent decades ago. The "Nexter" generation (born after 1980) is characterized as confident, achievement-oriented, tenacious, and optimistic (Zemke, 2001). However, this group may

166

be less independent than the previous age cohort, needing more supervision and structure (Brown, 2001). So, as these students enter nursing programs, faculty may need to help them understand what is required in the way of out-of-class preparation, provide detailed information about assignments, and clearly identify consequences of missing deadlines or being unprepared.

4. Expectations Unique to Nursing Faculty. In addition to the many roles and responsibilities common to all faculty, additional expectations are placed on nursing faculty. They often are expected to maintain clinical expertise, instruct students in clinical agencies, and engage in faculty practice. Moreover, nursing faculty who supervise students in clinical agencies may be responsible for an increasing number of very ill patients, adding an element not experienced by faculty in non-health care disciplines. Reflecting changing learning and work environments, nursing faculty are expected to develop proficiency in distance learning technology (AACN, 1999b; Potempa, 2001) and revise curricula to prepare graduates to excel in a rapidly changing health care environment (for example, see Tanner, 2001). The increase in mature students in accelerated programs adds the requirement to find challenging experiences for these students. What effect do these multiple roles, high expectations, and increased time commitments have upon the retention of nursing faculty and their ability to fully engage in an academic community? An AACN Issue Bulletin (1999a) on the faculty shortage asserts that faculty life "presents a harder road than private practice or administration" (p. 3). "The expectation on faculty to 'do it all' remains in many [nursing] schools and probably is a major reason for an unhappy and stressful work environment" (Rudy, 2001, p. 402). While further study of faculty workplace issues is needed, several authors report increased stress (Oermann, 1998), emotional exhaustion (Fong, 1993), burnout (Brendtro & Hegge, 2000; De Young & Bliss, 1995), and early retirement (AACN, 1999a) among nursing faculty.

H. Alternative Career Choices

Coupled with inadequate enrollment and graduations in master's and doctoral programs is a lack of preparation and possibly a perceived lack of interest in teaching. In 1976–1977, 24.7 percent of graduates from nursing master's programs were education (teaching) majors (National League for Nursing, 1988). By 1994, only 11.3 percent of graduates majored in education and in 2002 the percentage dropped to 3.5 percent (Berlin & Bednash, 1995; Berlin, Stennett, & Bednash, 2003a). This downward trend in nursing education majors was concomitant with increased emphasis on and interest in the nurse practitioner (NP) role, and since the mid-1990s, NP or combined NP/Clinical Nurse Specialist (CNS) enrollees and graduates have comprised the majority of master's enrollees and graduates. In 2002, 53.0 percent of master's enrollees and 60.1 percent of master's graduates were NP or combined NP/CNS majors (Berlin, Stennett, & Bednash, 2003a). These programs focus on preparing individuals for clinical practice and may not result in a large number of graduates pursuing doctoral education. Master's degree graduates prepared as NPs found an increasing number of employment opportunities in both ambulatory and hospital-based clinical practice (Hinshaw, 2001). Many of these positions offer a good match between graduates' values and skills and those of their prospective employers.

As noted previously, an increasing percentage of nursing doctoral recipients planned to be employed in settings other than nursing education (National Opinion Research Center, 2001). The primary interest of doctoral program graduates returning to or accepting their first academic appointments is the development of research programs. In some institutions it has been reported that few are interested in teaching, and even fewer are interested in teaching undergraduate students (AACN, 1999a). Although AACN supports doctoral preparation for the faculty role, half of current faculty hold master's degrees (Berlin, Stennett, & Bednash, 2003a). These individuals are invaluable faculty resources. However, "Until we have a faculty that is fully credentialed and contributing to all three aspects of our mission (teaching, research, and service), nursing programs will be vulnerable on campus, because the small numbers of doctorally prepared faculty de facto diminish contributions to the full mission of the institution" (Anderson, 1998, p. 6).

Section III: Short-Term Strategies for Expanding the Capacity of Current Faculty

Section II summarized issues related to the dwindling numbers of full-time faculty. The various challenges described offer nursing education a unique opportunity to develop and implement innovative, practical solutions in response to increasingly complex concerns, as nursing has done successfully throughout its history. The purpose of this section is to outline a variety of short-term strategies to alleviate the faculty shortage. It must be emphasized that many schools have developed exceptionally creative programs and initiatives that respond to current challenges and intercept future problems, including many of the suggestions included in this document. Others may find useful strategies described in this section, and as modeled by other schools. Clearly, not all of the strategies presented here are feasible in every setting, nor is this an exhaustive list. Institutions face different constraints and possibilities, depending on their demographic characteristics and geographic location. Each school is urged to engage in discussions with their own faculty, as well as with institutional, industry, and community leaders to seek location-specific opportunities to expand current faculty capacity.

1. ISSUE: Faculty capacity can be expanded in nontraditional ways with current resources.

Traditionally, nursing has objected to utilizing non-nurse faculty, recruiting nurse faculty with non-nursing degrees, and/or sharing resources and courses across disciplines and specialties, even though these non-traditional approaches may provide an important solution to a nursing faculty shortage and enhance student learning. The time has never been more appropriate to look for new approaches that make more sense. For example, nursing schools can create core courses that meet requirements across several specialty tracks. Interdisciplinary courses such as physical assessment, pharmacology, informatics, and gerontology can be developed on topics applicable to students representing a variety of health professions. Selected nursing classes/courses might be taught by non-nurse faculty, such as physicians, epidemiologists, statisticians, health policy analysts,

169

education specialists, and ethicists. Selected administrative positions might be held by well qualified non-nurses. For example, the Assistant Dean for the undergraduate program at Loyola University Chicago and Associate Dean for Research at the University of California, San Francisco are not nurses. While traditional "team teaching" may be labor intensive, sharing resources and developing joint initiatives among faculty and across programs, disciplines, departments, and even between universities can save money, spare limited faculty resources, and model a spirit of professional and interdisciplinary collaboration, a value that nursing espouses.

Adoption of a broader view of the educational requirements for nurse faculty status deserves special consideration. Advanced practice nurses and other nurses who are skilled in clinical practice, management, teaching, or research but who lack traditional academic preparation in nursing are an untapped resource for faculty. For example, according to data from the National Sample Survey of Registered Nurses, there are an estimated 3,000 advanced practice nurses who are nationally certified, and hold doctoral degrees, but do not hold a master's degree in nursing (Division of Nursing, 2001). Regardless of other credentials, the master's degree in nursing is required by some state regulatory bodies as a prerequisite for nursing faculty positions. This also affects students in some BSN to PhD programs that do not receive a master's degree. These students may be required to defer a teaching position until completing the doctorate. As long as these barriers exist, many expert clinicians—and potentially expert faculty—are prevented from teaching when they are needed most. Using these clinicians in creative faculty partnerships, with shared responsibility for courses, can expand faculty capacity.

Faculty recruitment might include previously untried outreach strategies. For example, pharmacy education is experiencing the same phenomenon of faculty shortfalls as nursing. For the past three years the American Association of Colleges of Pharmacy has sponsored a special session at an American Society of Health-System Pharmacists clinical meeting (American Association of Colleges of Pharmacy, 2003). The two-hour session, titled "Is an Academic Career in My Future?" has enjoyed increasing attendance over the years. The session includes several different speakers who candidly depict the faculty shortage, highlight the many positive aspects of an academic career, and offer specific advice on how to be successful as a faculty member. Similarly, the Medical College of Ohio offers a seminar for master's prepared nurses titled "Are You Interested in Getting a Doctoral Degree?" which includes a segment on academic careers (AACN, 2002c). Nurse educators host, plan, and attend an impressive number and variety of professional conferences and activities in their various professional capacities. Suggesting these types of programs to inform practicing nurses about and attract them to the faculty role may be a good investment. Other schools have developed master's programs that respond to the faculty shortage. The University of Arkansas for Medical Sciences prepares nurse educators in a federally funded master's program specifically designed to attract minority and disadvantaged students, particularly for utilization in underserved parts of the state (AACN, 2003b).

In addition to readily available sources of faculty described above, current approaches can be modified to increase the faculty pool. Traditional nursing programs may not be configured in ways that facilitate a clear and timely path to completion. For example, full-time employed nurses who desire to prepare for the faculty role on a part-time basis may face major impediments to this process. Employed nurses who attempt to combine part-time graduate study with full-time employment often face inflexible work schedules and increased clinical workloads imposed by employers because of the nursing shortage. San Francisco State University's cohort master's program was designed to facilitate the academic experience of working nurses, and has had the additional benefit of increasing the number of graduates accepting teaching positions and pursuing doctoral study (AACN, 2003a). Even though many schools of nursing have modified their graduate programs to make them more available to working students, periodic review of prerequisites, matriculation policies, and class scheduling may be in order to ensure that programs are not unduly exclusive or restrictive. Local nursing executives might be queried about the days their facilities are best staffed so that course days and times can be planned accordingly.

In a similar vein, many nurse educators continue to accept the traditional view that significant clinical experience as a registered nurse is essential before matriculating in a graduate program that prepares students for specialization and/or advanced practice. This position may not be accurate and is not supported in the empirical literature. It certainly bears scrutiny in the face of decreasing faculty resources. While high academic standards should not be compromised, rethinking any artificial eligibility criteria may be a useful strategy to increase enrollments in nursing graduate programs.

Not only should we reconsider the experience prerequisite for nurses seeking graduate education, we also should reconsider whether a nursing undergraduate degree is an essential prerequisite to graduate study in nursing. One excellent source of future faculty includes individuals who earned degrees in fields other than nursing. Second-degree or accelerated programs transition these individuals into nursing careers in streamlined ways and often in an abbreviated time frame. Although these programs are not new, they have proliferated over the past several years. In 1990, there were 31 baccalaureate and 12 master's programs designed for second-degree students (Bednash, Berlin, & Haux, 1991). By fall 2002, there were 105 baccalaureate and 34 master's programs in operation (Berlin, Stennett, & Bednash, 2003a). These individuals bring a wealth of academic ability, knowledge, and experience; plus they offer a different perspective to nursing, patient care, and the health care system (AACN, 2002a; Anderson, 2002). In short, these graduates may make excellent faculty members.

There is no question that nontraditional students pose unique challenges and require creativity and open-mindedness of faculty. We do not yet know if second-degree and accelerated programs are universally successful, and this is an important area of inquiry. One recent study (White, Wax, & Berrey, 2000) described a combined undergraduate and graduate nursing program designed primarily to prepare non-nurses with degrees in other fields for the nurse practitioner (NP) role. The program took roughly three years to complete, consistent with other accelerated master's programs across the country (AACN, 2002a). Twenty-nine graduates participated in the study, answering questions about their experiences. Of the 23 graduates employed as NPs, the majority believed the educational program prepared them adequately for the advanced practice role, attributing this largely to excellent clinical experiences and assignments. Interestingly, the majority did not believe that experience as a registered nurse was necessary to function in the NP role, although many had nursing experience. (The program encouraged all students to work as staff nurses when they became eligible, and 19 had done so.) This illustrates that programs can be designed to provide adequate basic as well as advanced clinical experiences for second-degree or accelerated students. Unfortunately, the authors stated that the graduates' "most commonly mentioned challenges included resistance from nurses, NPs, and traditional students who held the belief that the nontraditional students had not 'paid their dues' the traditional way" (p. 220). Nurse educators may know colleagues who hold similar views and who need encouragement to try non-traditional approaches in these challenging times.

The use of technology can provide additional immediate solutions to increase the capacity of faculty to support education, research, and practice. The growing importance of distance technology, and in particular, Web-based media to deliver educational course work is evident, and it is revolutionizing higher education. However, well-designed distance education programs require long-term planning and considerable institutional financial investment in equipment, support services, and faculty development (AACN, 1999b). Collaboration with existing distance programs may offer a faculty-sparing effect for selected courses.

Strategies:
1. Consolidate core curriculum requirements across nursing majors or clinical tracks to reduce duplication of faculty effort.
2. Accept courses from other disciplines as appropriate to meet nursing program requirements.
3. Develop joint academic activities with other disciplines (health care and non–health care) both within the university and among universities to capitalize on existing resources.

4. Create interprofessional courses to meet the common needs of multiple related disciplines.
5. Utilize expert non-nurse faculty to teach selected nursing classes/courses.
6. Utilize qualified non-nurse faculty to hold administrative positions within the nursing academic unit.
7. Identify any existing regulatory requirements that limit nurses with non-nursing graduate degrees from teaching in nursing programs so that efforts to remove these barriers can be planned.
8. Utilize the expertise of junior faculty by partnering them with senior, fully qualified faculty who can provide course oversight and faculty support without requiring the more labor-intensive team teaching.
9. Seek opportunities to sponsor educational sessions that inform nurses outside the academic setting about an academic career, emphasize the positive aspects of the role, and offer specific strategies for gaining the necessary credentials/experience to become faculty members.
10. As they exist, consider reducing or eliminating experience or other artificial prerequisites for graduate study.
11. Examine current curricula/programs and streamline them as much as possible to facilitate more timely program completion.
12. Remove impediments to graduate study for working nurses, such as offering more convenient times for courses, encouraging partnering institutions to offer students more flexible work schedules to accommodate class schedules, and offering courses specifically for partnering health care facilities, possibly at their site(s).
13. Attract more second-degree students to the nursing profession and encourage these and other high-achieving students to consider the faculty role early in their education.
14. Explore collaboration with schools or regional consortia that have successful distance education programs in place.

2. ISSUE: Retirement often has been viewed as an all-or-none phenomenon in the academic nursing community, making an

experienced pool of faculty unavailable for continued contributions to the nursing academic unit.

Most nursing faculty members retire between the ages of 61.5 and 62.5 years (AACN, 1993, 1994, 2002b). Many faculty approaching retirement would like to continue teaching in some capacity, but may be unable to do so because of restrictive university policies and/or retirement plan provisions. Rather than retirement marking the end of professional productivity, as many as half of retiring American academics return to the workforce (Dorfman, 1989). Research (Kelly & Swisher, 1998) has shown that, although retirement often is welcomed by nurses and valued as a time to focus on the self, retirees nevertheless miss professional affiliations and the discipline of going to work. Women seem to have more difficulty retiring than men and are more reluctant to retire. In fact, work may be more important in the lives of older women than previously recognized in the literature. While retirement is viewed as an attractive option to those whose work roles and environments are perceived as stressful and not enjoyable, many retiring nurses actively seek opportunities to volunteer and otherwise stay busy. These observations have particular implications for the female-dominated nursing profession, especially the subgroup of aging nurse academicians who might remain active if allowed and encouraged to do so.

AACN's 2002 survey of resignations and retirements indicated that of the 161 retirees, 10 (6.2%) are continuing to teach on a part-time basis (AACN, 2002b). Some colleges and universities are recognizing the value of retired scholars and are creating ways to keep them involved in the academic community. For example, Emory University has created an Emeritus College comprised of retired professors across disciplines. They meet for monthly meals and intellectual activities, teach selected classes, and participate in organized programs that keep them active in the lives of students (Fogg, 2003). The University of Southern California's Emeriti Center offers modest research stipends to retired faculty, recognizes them for continuing scholarship, and supports an off-campus lecture series in which they speak at functions in the community.

Retirement policies have been reconsidered at some institutions to allow retired faculty to return to teaching responsibilities. For example, the University of California (including their two schools of nursing at San Francisco and Los Angeles) have a faculty recall policy that allows faculty to collect their full retirement (which may be as high as 100% of their salary depending on years of service) while being paid for additional faculty service in teaching or administration. The policy demands that faculty be retired for a minimum of 30 days and be recalled for 47% time or less. The University of Florida-Gainesville also enables colleges to hire retired faculty members as soon as one month following their retirement date. The retired faculty member is not eligible for benefits and is restricted in the amount of income that can be earned each year for their services if they are to continue to collect retirement income. Nursing may do well to utilize these and similar ideas to encourage retiring and retired faculty to remain active in the full array of nursing education activities.

Strategies:

1. Examine college/university retirement policies and work to eliminate unnecessary restrictions to continued faculty service, particularly mandatory retirement ages and financial penalties for retired faculty who return to work.
2. Design new phased retirement plans that support the inclusion of productive retired faculty.
3. Redesign current faculty workload to accommodate part-time retired faculty.
4. If monetary compensation is problematic, reward retired faculty with incentives such as reimbursement for conferences, assignment of a graduate assistant, and release time for professional activities rather than direct salary support.
5. In addition to teaching, consider other ways that qualified retired faculty might save current faculty time by counseling or tutoring students, supervising in skills labs, mentoring students and/or faculty, assisting with research projects, and serving as ambassadors to the community.

6. As an inducement to participation, create programs that formally include and recognize retired nursing faculty as a continuing, productive part of the nursing academic unit.
7. Cultivate a workplace that is perceived by faculty as positive, productive, enriching, and satisfying so that they will be enticed to continue employment longer than originally planned.

3. ISSUE: Nursing clinical education is resource-intensive for colleges and universities, but is critically important for the safe teaching of nursing as a practice discipline.

Nursing clinical instruction as practiced today is expensive in that it traditionally has been accomplished in small groups of students with close supervision because the learning experience includes assuming responsibility for direct patient care. In addition, faculty must have education and expertise in the specific specialty area in which they supervise students. Therefore, even schools with small student enrollment require multiple faculty experts to represent applicable specialties and to directly supervise learners as they provide care to human beings. Nursing educators are becoming increasingly creative in offering high quality clinical experiences to students in the face of decreasing faculty resources. Many schools have developed formal partnerships with clinical facilities to use expert clinicians to teach students and thereby increase faculty capacity. These partnerships have varying characteristics and incentives. Some partnerships yield direct financial benefits to one or both partners, while others have indirect benefits. For example, non-salaried faculty appointments often are offered to agency clinicians who serve as teachers and/or clinical preceptors for students. Individuals selected for these roles enjoy increased professional recognition and other indirect rewards. In return for providing clinical teachers/preceptors, the agency may benefit from faculty services such as teaching or consultation; preferred placement of employees in the academic program; the benefit of collaboration as they seek magnet recognition and similar status from external agencies; and priority in recruiting the school's students upon graduation. These creative and mutually beneficial relationships are time-consuming and labor-intensive to develop and require much thought about the benefits to be derived by each partner. However, these types of professional relationships may be a key to future success in nursing clinical education as faculty losses continue.

A large number of AACN member schools have created formal partnerships with their health service colleagues to increase nursing enrollments (undergraduate and graduate) and/or expand faculty capacity. For example, partnerships at the University of New Mexico and University of Iowa derive significant benefits to both partners, and have been highlighted at AACN conferences (AACN, 2002d, 2003c), but other examples abound. Initiatives by the University of Florida, the University of South Florida, and the University of Virginia, among others, specifically increase clinical faculty capacity and improve the learning experience of students (AACN, 2002c, 2003b). The University of California, San Francisco–affiliated university medical centers provide three-year scholarships to students in the masters-entry program in nursing if students promise to work full time for one year between achieving their registered nurse license (earned after one year in the program) and returning to school. Students also promise to work at the institution part-time while continuing in the master's program. Loma Linda University's partnering hospital encourages experienced clinicians to supervise students by paying preceptors a slightly higher salary (AACN, 2002c). Numerous nursing schools host programs to benefit the hospital clinicians who supervise students. For example, Emory University hosts an Annual Preceptor Institute to address clinical topics of interest (AACN, 2002c). Carson-Newman College specifically prepares agency preceptors for their critically important role in evaluating students (AACN, 2003a).

Partnerships between clinical facilities and academic programs offer the additional benefit of engaging both partners in discussion about how nursing is practiced in the real world and how it should be taught. Nursing programs consistently have not sought this expert advice from service colleagues. Dr. Tim Porter-O'Grady (2001), who often consults with health care facilities, asserts that nursing is changing quickly from practice-based activities such as "bathing, treating, changing, feeding, intervening, drugging, and discharging" to knowledge-based activities of "accessing, informing, guiding, teaching, counseling, typing, and linking. . ." (p. 183). Dr. Barbara Mark on the faculty at the University of North Carolina at Chapel Hill is engaged in funded research dedicated to redesigning the work of nursing. She states "We need to figure out how to redesign the work of nursing to get maximum efficiency and maximum effectiveness from the nurses we have" rather than simply adding more nurses (Vickers, 2002, p.6). During these times of possibly dramatic transitions in what constitutes nursing, formal collaboration between service and education will better identify emerging clinical issues, analyze actual roles and expectations of practicing nurses, and develop the required nursing curriculum.

In addition to looking internally, nursing may benefit from examining curricular designs, models, and teaching strategies from other health disciplines that offer effective learning and require fewer clinical faculty, such as expanded use of non-faculty clinical preceptors, concentrated clinical experience (e.g., 40 hours/week) late in the program, and increased use of simulations in the clinical laboratory in lieu of patient care assignments. Nursing traditionally has valued and even required one model for teaching: integrated theory and small group, faculty-supervised clinical practice throughout the nursing program. However, little empirical evidence exists to validate these preferred approaches as best practices in nursing clinical education. Nursing must be open to a variety of clinical teaching models that may have a faculty-sparing effect.

Strategies:

1. Increase formal partnerships between schools of nursing and clinical facilities, identifying and capitalizing on specific benefits that are attractive and useful to both partners.
2. Develop clinical faculty appointments or other forms of recognition/inducement to qualified clinical agency personnel in return for their supervising/teaching students in those agencies.
3. As needed, educate agency personnel regarding strategies for clinical teaching and evaluation.

4. Include appropriate clinical agency personnel on school of nursing committees and task forces to gain their pragmatic perspective on the education of students.
5. Import clinical education strategies from other health disciplines, both internal and external to one's own setting, that demonstrate a faculty-sparing effect.
6. Explore use of virtual reality/simulated clinical experiences in supervised learning resource centers to reduce demands on clinical faculty.

4. ISSUE: We have insufficient evidence regarding how to best utilize faculty and need more educational research.

Nursing has a long, proud tradition of excellence in education, often leading the way for other disciplines. This has never been more apparent than now, when the profession boasts an impressive number and variety of programs and periodicals devoted to nursing education. However, the overall decline in master's enrollments and increased emphasis on clinical specialization at the master's level in the past two decades help explain the lower number of nursing master's students specializing in education. Further, the decline in doctoral graduations, and the relatively small percentage of doctorally prepared nurses who choose an academic career may adversely affect the amount and variety of educational research being conducted. For example, the traditional clinical teaching model of one instructor for a small group of students and specific faculty-to-student ratios (e.g., 1:6; 1:8) mandated in many states developed out of practices deemed suitable at the time, but which may no longer be most appropriate. For the most part, these models and ratios have not been tested.

Faculty often approach didactic and clinical teaching the way *they* were taught, rather than incorporating new techniques based on educational research findings that may have direct impact on faculty productivity/capacity and optimal student learning. Therefore, we need to establish best practices in nursing education that are based on empirical evidence. Furthermore, with nursing and health care in a state of rapid change and faculty resources rapidly declining, nursing does not have the luxury of approaching teaching with traditional labor-intensive or trial-and-error approaches. We need specific research that validates best teaching practices in order to maximize our teaching resources.

The scholarship of teaching is a recognized part of the full range of scholarship within the discipline of nursing (AACN, 1999c). However, there may be a tendency to place higher value on the scholarship of clinical practice, and the considerable resources of the National Institutes of Health are not available to faculty who want to test innovative educational programs. Therefore, in some instances, faculty who are dedicated to conducting educational research to help develop a science of teaching may struggle for recognition of their work and may have difficulty obtaining funding or promotion.

Strategies:

1. Work with nursing academic colleagues to emphasize the legitimacy and importance of educational research to the future of nursing.
2. Conduct research to better understand the phenomena of teaching and learning and to document the effects of various educational strategies.
3. Where necessary, study any specified faculty-to-student ratios that do not make sense in the current educational context, assess their origin, and consider their continued applicability.
4. Study existing nontraditional/accelerated programs to determine their success, lessons learned, and potential use as models for future programs.
5. Seek funding from organizations that focus on the scholarship of teaching, such as the Carnegie Foundation for the Advancement of Teaching and Learning.
6. Draw upon the expertise and seek collaboration with organizations/entities that focus on educational research.

5. ISSUE: Faculty require professional development, mentoring, and institutional encouragement to master the faculty role and continue in it.

As mentioned in Section 2, the college/university environment is changing in dramatic ways, adapting to the demands of the information age, reexamining what and how students learn, and responding to increasingly varied and demanding learners and new workforce skills (Berberet & McMillin, 2002). This can be positive and exhilarating; one of the most highly valued aspects of the job. The demanding educational environment and the full array of role expectations encourage faculty to embrace a constant state of self-improvement in order to be fully successful.

One of the most crucial expectations of faculty is to understand learning and to apply that knowledge in determining both what to teach and how to teach. Hopefully, most faculty have realized that the current higher education environment is about the learner and learning rather than the teacher and teaching. Educators now are expected to facilitate learning rather than convey vast amounts of content (Porter-O'Grady, 2001; Berberet & McMillin, 2002). In nursing, clinical expertise is essential to professional success, but clinical proficiency alone is not sufficient to convey nursing knowledge and practice to others in a meaningful, useful, appropriate way. Excellent nurses are not necessarily expert teachers. Because of the explosion of information on the art and science of teaching adults, faculty members cannot hope to be completely successful in their teaching without formal mechanisms of professional development. Without this instruction and support, a new faculty member may receive negative student evaluations, become frustrated with the faculty role, and seek other employment opportunities. Even experienced faculty can benefit from regular faculty development, particularly as new educational research and strategies are introduced that can improve their teaching. Doctoral programs in nursing may wish to add required education content and/or mentoring opportunities to familiarize all students with the academic role.

Strong orientation programs and ongoing faculty development opportunities are pivotal to keeping all faculty informed and confident about the teaching aspect of their role. These activities may occur in individual classes, formal courses, or independent activities. They may consist of informal peer mentoring such as the program used successfully in academic medicine (Pololi, Knight, Dennis, & Frankel, 2002), or it may be an intangible element that is nurtured in a community of teachers seeking to improve their expertise (Diekelman, 2002). They may be based on interdisciplinary national initiatives such as the Carnegie Academy for the Scholarship of Teaching and Learning (CASTL) Higher Education Program (Carnegie Foundation for the Advancement of Teaching, 2003) and the Preparing Future Faculty Program (Preparing Future Faculty National Office, 2003). Emory University's Clinical Teaching Institute has the goal of increased teaching competence and inclusion of clinical experts in the teaching of students and enjoys the additional benefit of recruiting new faculty (AACN, 2002c). Faculty can take advantage of a myriad of formal education programs, including the on-line master's level concentration in education such as that offered by Saint Joseph's College of Maine, one of the most heavily enrolled specialty tracks in education among AACN member schools. In addition, faculty can avail themselves of the new modular on-line Education Scholar Program (2003) endorsed by AACN. Whatever faculty development approach is adopted, it is imperative that formal assistance be offered to faculty, both as they begin the new role and as they continue to master it throughout their careers.

In addition to conveying important information on teaching and learning, faculty development activities can help nurse educators become more comfortable with other aspects of their roles (scholarship, service, and other university missions), minimizing their struggle with the sometimes conflicting expectations. The full academic role has been described in the literature (Billings, 2003). Educators value being part of the academic community. "At the same time, however, faculty members express frustration with new responsibilities that bring differing and sometimes conflicting expectations and demands that leave many of them feeling stretched beyond reasonable bounds" (Berberet & McMillin, p. 9). In addition to informing faculty about their various roles, it is time to reconsider what tasks are pivotal to the faculty role, and which are less important. Can some traditional tasks and responsibilities be eliminated or relinquished? Can others be modified, transferred, or shared? Other disciplines are engaged in this type of self-analysis. A Minnesota medical school faculty examined their shared expectations, identified areas of strength and weakness as a group, prioritized their roles according to current information about their productivity and vitality, and identified areas that might be improved by faculty development activities or informal mentoring (Bland, Seaquist, Pacala, Center, & Finstad, 2002). As a part of the national Faculty Workload Project, Ithaca College of New York embarked on an effort to systematically reconfigure faculty work assignments appropriate to their discipline and educational goals. Seven departments, including physical therapy, encouraged faculty to explore innovative teaching-learning models, consolidate or streamline the curriculum, and increase the use of nontraditional environments and technologies in learning. After one year, both student and faculty satisfaction were increased as a result of changes instituted, and these changes will be used to create a college-wide model for revising faculty work (Association of Governing Boards, 2002).

Encouraging and facilitating master's prepared nursing faculty to pursue the doctoral degree is the ultimate in faculty development and often can be done without losing the faculty asset. For example, faculty may opt to pursue on-line nursing doctoral degrees such as those offered by Duquesne University, University of Arizona, and University of the Wisconsin–Milwaukee, or summers-only nursing doctoral programs such as those offered by Loyola University Chicago and Catholic University of America. Other programs, such as University of Colorado, offer combinations of intensive and on-line courses particularly useful for those who do not live nearby.

Strategies:

1. Develop an AACN Essentials of the Nursing Professoriate document to describe the complexity of the faculty role and guide faculty development efforts of individual schools as well as programmatic activities of AACN.
2. Identify minimum faculty development activities that should be required of all faculty, and incorporate these into internal hiring and/or evaluation strategies.
3. Formally orient part-time and adjunct faculty to their roles, keep them up-to-date on school and course expectations, and offer guidance and development as required.

4. Critically evaluate what faculty roles, tasks, and expectations can be eliminated or modified, and how faculty talents can be best utilized.

5. Provide faculty with a wide variety of role development opportunities, such as college/university-based activities, local and national conferences (including AACN conferences), and national programs such as the Web-based Education Scholar program, as endorsed by AACN.

6. Encourage faculty to complete post-master's or post-doctoral certificate programs in education for those who are not academically prepared in nursing education.

7. Cultivate an academic climate that offers guidance, encouragement, mentoring, discussion, resources, and other role development opportunities for all faculty members.

8. Incorporate nursing education content in all nursing doctoral programs in order to make doctoral students aware of this important and attractive career option.

9. In all settings and with all audiences, portray nursing and nursing education as scholarly and desirable careers.

10. Encourage master's prepared nursing faculty to pursue continued faculty service, and support them in pursuit of doctoral education.

Section IV. Long-Term Strategies for Expanding the Future Pool of Nursing Faculty

Although short-term strategies may address immediate needs for faculty in schools of nursing, long-term solutions are required to meet the combined challenge of depleted faculty ranks and the escalating need for nurses. The current and projected shortage of faculty is complex and multifactorial. Ultimately, solutions must also be complex and multifactorial, with appropriate long-term strategies.

A. Recruitment

1. Develop a positive message. The declining number of those completing nursing graduate programs combined with a similar decline in colleagues who are joining academic communities is troublesome. Developing and articulating a positive message about the value of nursing higher education and an academic career is a first step in recruiting new academic colleagues. All nurses, particularly academicians, can deliver a positive message by serving as role models in all settings. In addition, promotion of clinical nursing leadership with emphasis on intellectual skills and practice autonomy will highlight nursing as an attractive career choice for students, many of whom later may be recruited into faculty positions. As a whole, those who have chosen a nursing academic career perceive it as a rewarding and satisfying career choice. They have numerous opportunities to identify the specific aspects of the career that make it attractive. Hosting information sessions and similar activities devoted to attracting qualified nurses to the faculty or to graduate study offer both short- and long-term benefits. A positive message about nursing education as a career choice should be conveyed to both nursing and external audiences.

2. Recruit at younger ages. The mean age of the faculty in schools of nursing must be decreased. The most obvious strategy is recruiting younger people into academics. Efforts must be made to increase the future pool of faculty by focusing on the decision-making process of middle and high school students. Large scale advertising campaigns such as Nurses for a Healthier Tomorrow (2000) and the Johnson & Johnson (2002) Campaign for Nursing's Future are making strides at the national level. Locally, nursing schools can sponsor educational and social activities at middle and high schools in their areas, using these occasions to highlight the positive aspects of nursing and academic career choices. For example, today's young people are drawn toward careers that require intelligence, encourage autonomy, and utilize technology. Many are attracted to medicine and science as disciplines that appear to best utilize their talents. An effective message to them will emphasize that a nursing career utilizes the very qualities and skills they value. Further, nurse educators can inform middle and high school guidance counselors about the modern roles of professional nurses; help them recognize and overcome gender and occupational stereotypes; and emphasize

186

the rigorous nature of nursing education so these counselors can encourage qualified young people toward a nursing, and possibly academic nursing, career.

A number of nursing programs have instituted these types of recruiting programs in their communities (Health Resources and Services Administration, 2001; AACN, 2003a). For example, Hampton University begins marketing nursing as a career to elementary schools in their community. For over a decade, the University of California, Los Angeles, has hosted 7th and 8th graders from an inner city school at a two-week summer program where they learn about health care, work with nurse researchers, and meet students and faculty. The University of Arkansas for Medical Sciences has recruiting initiatives targeted at middle and high schools as well as feeder colleges in the state. Loma Linda University, University of Akron, and Cedarville University have projects aimed at helping pre-nursing and nursing students overcome academic and other barriers to success in school. Many other university schools of nursing have outreach programs designed to attract elementary and high school students to nursing. Because these programs are heavily invested with faculty, students are able to see the strengths of both faculty and nursing roles, achieving two important purposes. Partnerships between high school districts and college/university faculty provide important internships and mentorships that can increase enrollees for little cost. During college, there are additional strategic opportunities to encourage the consideration of nursing academics as a career. This is particularly true for students who have not selected a major, and in some cases for those who are unsure about the field they have chosen. For example, young people with education majors and other health-related specialties can be encouraged to consider nursing (and ultimately academics) as a career choice. The choice of nursing can be supported by developing matriculation agreements across colleges.

3. Seamless basic and advanced nursing preparation. Methods to streamline the trajectory from basic nursing education to academics must be explored and strengthened, even if it means restructuring current systems and cultures. As previously mentioned, the cultural norm of requiring several years of clinical practice between undergraduate and graduate degrees prior to assuming a faculty role still is held by many nursing faculty. Movement from undergraduate to graduate programs must be easy and seamless for qualified students, so they can assume faculty positions more quickly. For example, a baccalaureate to master's/doctoral program may be initiated wherein a student admitted to a baccalaureate program would provisionally be admitted to a graduate program at the same time. By streamlining and accelerating progression through graduate education programs, we may attract younger students who don't bring significant financial and family responsibilities to their graduate experience; who can work part-time and study full-time rather than vice versa. Schools of nursing must find the delicate balance between attracting working nurses and encouraging timely completion of degrees.

4. Seek sources of financial aid. A cornerstone consideration in recruitment efforts must be financial aid. This aid could take several forms. The most obvious is improved financial aid for tuition and books. But more importantly for graduate students, financial aid also must include remuneration for lost pay while attending school. This financial assistance could take the form of outright grants to loans that are forgiven for a certain number of years of teaching service.

5. Support students from admission to graduation. The drop-out rate in undergraduate and graduate schools also must be addressed. Current students who struggle in both undergraduate and graduate nursing programs should be aggressively mentored and tutored, utilizing services of the university and community more so than intense nursing faculty resources. Data are now available that help faculty admission committees identify students who are most likely to complete programs successfully and in a timely manner (University of California, 2001). These data should be employed to inform admission requirements. Standardized screening and progression tools can be used in admission and continuation decisions in order to maximize student success. However, nursing must not increase its exclusivity during a time of severe shortage.

188

B. Retention

1. Enhance the work environment. Once faculty are recruited, all efforts must turn toward retention. One obvious strategy is to make the job more attractive by providing better salaries and benefits (especially at entry-level assistant professorships), lower faculty/student ratios, more autonomy, and better merit/reward systems. These measures require heavy support from state legislators (for publicly funded schools) and private industry or patrons (for private schools). Many deans and administrators have recognized these challenges and have been creative in finding ways to make faculty positions attractive, particularly by developing academic tracks in which teaching excellence is rewarded.

2. Support faculty. Formal development and mentorship programs for new faculty and recently graduated doctoral students can reduce the frustrations that often accompany the transition into the faculty role. In addition, institutions might consider the establishment of "Academies of Nurse Educators," with the goal of elevating the teaching role through the support of a core group of talented teachers who will, in turn, improve the environment for all teaching faculty and serve as models and mentors for other faculty. Strategies to support beginning researchers also must be addressed, both by the federal government and by universities. These strategies must include financial support for beginning researchers, effective mentorship programs to insure success in the academic role, and adjusted teaching and university service to allow junior faculty the time they need to build careers.

C. Collaboration

1. In the local community. Resources to implement various strategies to enhance faculty recruitment will require a multi-level approach. Legislative liaisons are essential. For example, state legislatures are the source of funding critical to many schools. Academic leaders must become increasingly knowledgeable about legislative solutions and resources and must devote time to developing and maintaining these vital relationships. As the scope of nursing practice changes and the nursing and faculty shortages increase, state nursing groups may need to assertively reconsider nurse practice acts and accreditation or regulatory requirements that limit timely and creative approaches to resolving current problems. Partnerships with high schools and community colleges, private industry, health care providers and insurers, current faculty, and other stakeholders must be pursued to seek broad-based solutions and solicit money and other resources. Schools of nursing may have to collaborate with each other to augment rather than duplicate each other's strengths. Multiple governmental agencies should be explored as important sources of funding, such as the Centers for Disease Control and Prevention or the Department of Health and Human Services. A strong willingness to explore unconventional alternatives is required.

2. With other disciplines. Collaboration with other disciplines can provide increased faculty resources for students. Health care is increasingly complex and, by its very nature, interdisciplinary. Yet most schools do not provide students with an early introduction to the other disciplines. Interdisciplinary collaboration across the professions in required courses and clinical rotations would not only provide a partial solution to the nursing faculty shortage but also would provide students an opportunity to develop the attitudes and skills required for effective collaboration.

3. With other professional organizations. AACN has long been engaged in collaborative work with other national professional associations and organizations that have a stake in the future of nursing and nursing education. These affiliations and collaborations with educational and service entities must continue, because the issues we face are complex and interactive. For example, the nursing faculty shortage is a significant element of the larger nursing shortage. Nursing faculty issues are a subset of faculty issues for all disciplines. Changes in nursing practice directly affect nursing education. The issues concerning nursing education for the profession are issues of importance to *all* nurses. As a result, our concerns and spheres of influence overlap, and problems must continue to be resolved in a collaborative way.

Developing a "positive message" about a nursing academic career is a good example of potential collaboration across disciplines. Nursing education and the faculty shortage are of concern to multiple professional groups and nurses at all levels. The faculty shortage, like the nursing shortage, affects all stakeholders and will require support from all interested parties.

   4. Within AACN. As previously mentioned, an AACN document describing the Essentials of the Nursing Professoriate would meet an immediate need to specifically describe elements of the faculty role. This document would be a useful reference as schools and AACN develop faculty development programs and initiatives in the immediate future. Further, it would form the basis for refinement and expansion as nursing practice changes and nursing education must respond accordingly in the future. In addition, AACN may want to more fully investigate specific issues that may have an impact on the faculty shortage. AACN member schools are an excellent source of information about the direction the association should go to meet the challenges of the faculty shortage.

In Summary

Nursing education has had a long and successful history and often leads other disciplines in educational research, innovative teaching-learning activities, and problem resolution in the academic environment. The faculty shortage offers nurse educators an unparalleled opportunity to challenge past norms and think collaboratively and nontraditionally to meet the future. Nursing education may be shaped in new and exciting ways by the solutions developed to meet the current and future faculty shortage.

Appendix

This appendix stems from sessions at the AACN Hot Issues Conference, *Building Faculty Leadership During the Crisis: Solutions from a Faculty Perspective,* held April 24–26, 2003, in San Antonio, Texas. The conference took place immediately after the initial release of the Task Force on Future Faculty's white paper, and the paper was showcased during a program session.

Discussion during both that session and the closing session offered excellent examples of what member schools are doing to ameliorate the faculty shortage.

AACN Task Force on Future Faculty Program Session from AACN Hot Issues Conference, Friday, April 25, 2003, San Antonio, Texas

Facilitated by Sheila Haas, PhD, RN, FAAN, Dean, Niehoff School of Nursing, Loyola University Chicago Task Force Member

Short-Term Strategies

- University of the Incarnate Word recruits underrepresented nurses into faculty roles. Four minority RN to BSN students are funded with state tobacco settlement money plus a student employment budget to work part-time with a faculty mentor in all aspects of the faculty role. They receive a tuition-free master's degree immediately after completing the BSN. On master's graduation, they agree to work in a faculty position for two years. This initiative has the added benefit of energizing the faculty working with these students.
- California State University Long Beach works closely with the nurse executive at a local hospital on a number of initiatives. The nursing executive serves on the school's advisory board and is integral to the program. At the hospital's request, the school has on-site BSN and master's programs for hospital employees as a recruiting and retention strategy. The CNS graduate program has been revived specifically for the hospital. Faculty teach the on-site courses on an overload basis, earning a fee in addition to their full-time salary. The school is working with the hospital in their application for magnet status. The hospital has furnished the school with a faculty position to increase the number of generic students.
- Seattle University works with the local Veteran's Affairs hospital chief nurse executive. The hospital donated a master's-prepared nurse to enable students to perform clinical hours there.
- The University of Texas El Paso receives both subsidized faculty and cash for administrative costs and supplies from their clinical agency.

- New Mexico legislature recently passed a bill to allow state retirees to return to the state workforce, collect a full-time salary, and pause any retirement annuity to resume later. One retired nurse was enticed to return to the faculty full-time.
- Several states allow instructor-to-student ratio of 1:12 in clinical courses utilizing qualified preceptors, thereby expanding faculty capacity. Other states allow a 1:20 ratio (Delaware) or 1:25 (Texas) for precepted courses.
- Concern was expressed about recruiting part-time instructors to fill "holes" for a particular semester, with generous incentives based on urgent need. Full-time faculty who carry much responsibility over time may be resentful of inducements offered to these professionals.

Long-Term Strategies

- Numerous schools of nursing focus on recruiting high school students, but others believe that outreach to elementary and middle schools is necessary to engage student interest and ensure that students take the required math and science courses in high school. Loyola University Chicago sponsors nurse-managed school-based clinics as one way to make the nursing role visible and attractive to students. Guidance counselors are another valuable group to reach in order to educate students about nursing.
- West Virginia University developed a recruitment CD for counselors in middle and high schools to educate them about nursing. They also give a list of all nursing schools in the state to qualified applicants who cannot be accommodated.
- Illinois deans do something similar when a school cannot accept qualified applicants. The applicants are referred, sometimes individually by the dean, to other schools.
- The dean of Loyola University Chicago invites local chief nurse executives to semiannual breakfast meetings to determine if the school's graduates are meeting their respective agency's needs. In addition to helpful discussion among participants, these meetings generate useful ideas to take to the Board of Nursing and legislature.
- A dilemma was articulated regarding faculty recruitment. How do you recruit exceptional nurses as faculty while being honest

about the heavy workload and the salary level that often falls below what nurses could make in other roles? Finding the right message is critical. For example, a nine-month contract may be attractive to a nursing faculty member interested in working in another capacity during their three months away from the academic setting.

• The University of Minnesota encourages all colleges of nursing in the state to identify their top undergraduate students and then invites these students to attend a reception and learn more about doctoral education. This event is perceived as a reward for students.

Re-Thinking the Faculty "To-Do" List

Closing Program Session from AACN Hot Issues Conference, Saturday, April 26, 2003, San Antonio, Texas
Facilitated by Carole Anderson, PhD, RN, FAAN, Vice Provost for Academic Administration, The Ohio State University, Columbus, Ohio; Dorothy Powell, EdD, RN, FAAN, Associate dean for nursing, Howard University, Washington, D.C.
WORKLOAD (schools identified when known)

• Develop a revised notion of team teaching: "Turn Teaching." This technique is more efficient if instructors divide course workload and attend only their own classes rather than the traditional, labor-intensive model of team teaching in which all instructors participate in all course activities. One faculty might have full responsibility for a course "on paper" and other faculty have a fraction of the workload. *Advantages:* Students have the benefit of multiple instructors; instructors save time; instructors can trade off responsibility to allow team colleagues protected "scholarship time" for writing grants, attending conferences, etc. (University of Maryland); *Disadvantages:* Instructor may not have the faculty development opportunity of total responsibility for a course from beginning to end.

• As possible, delete responsibilities from the faculty role, such as advising, administration, and even committee work. Where is nursing faculty input critical?

- Save time and boost efficiency by improving faculty skills in meeting management, process improvement, and decision making. Consensus is not always possible. Vote and get over it!
- Different instructors teaching different sections of the same course do not need identical assignments. This saves faculty time by not having to meet, negotiate, and reach consensus. Different faculty expectations/assignments are not intrinsically unfair to students.
- Utilize different course numbers for lecture and clinical sections. One instructor coordinates the class and takes one clinical section; other instructors each take a clinical section. Team meetings are held at the beginning and end of each semester as necessary.
- Delineate work categories and assign faculty according to their particular strengths, i.e., classroom teaching, clinical teaching, research. What do people do best? An instructor with a lighter research load might assume a larger teaching load. An egalitarian philosophy that all faculty should be doing the same things is difficult to maintain. Concurrently, schools should mentor faculty in all aspects of the role so they can assume all required aspects of the role.
- University of Wisconsin–Madison has a Teaching Academy that encourages campus-wide emphasis on excellence in teaching at the undergraduate level. Master teachers are used as consultants, mentors, and peer evaluators. Doesn't include clinical instruction unique to nursing; a Summer Institute (also University of Wisconsin–Madison) offers selected faculty a paid five-day retreat to develop a specific project in June immediately after the semester ends. The application process requires description of the project and resources that will be required at the retreat. A team can apply to do a team project. On campuses where similar opportunities are not available, nursing may need to open a dialogue to see what other disciplines do well and what might be useful for nursing (e.g., increased use of simulation in engineering) or develop a multidisciplinary retreat on best practices.

ENVIRONMENT—How do we create a positive, collaborative environment that will encourage faculty to stay and entice graduate students to pursue an academic career?

- Collaborate with other schools that have a particular strength, not just with service institutions. For instance, the Howard and Yale Research Scholars Program offers selected Howard students the opportunity to participate in six weeks of intensive research at Yale and continue a project throughout the academic year at home. Programs such as these socialize students to roles we want them to assume in the future. (Howard University, Washington, DC)
- Use exceptional undergraduate students as Teaching Assistants in labs. Encourage those interested in teaching to take a graduate-level course while still at the undergraduate level.
- Saginaw Valley State University nursing faculty has adopted a "co-learners" philosophy with several innovative characteristics: teaching-learning experiences (no lectures are given; papers are combined with other experiences); changed terminology (term clinical [implies hospital setting] has been replaced with practicum [refers to all settings]); courses, for example, are named Critical Thinking I and II rather than Med-Surg I and II; instructors and students jointly determine norms at the beginning of each semester, by which all are expected to abide, such as sharing mistakes openly as learning opportunities, emphasis on self-reflection, etc.; changes were instituted after two summers of intense negotiation because faculty decided that they wanted to escape the medical model and replace it with something unique.
- Recognize that some faculty members are not suited to a particular setting. For instance, one who loves teaching may not be best suited to a research-intensive school because of the role expectations. An unhappy faculty member can "poison the well" and may need encouragement to consider other employment.
- *Have fun* in the work setting. Dress up on Halloween and award prizes for costumes. Laugh in faculty meetings. Sponsor social activities. Improve communication among faculty.

Give credit where it is due. Recognize contributions and successes of colleagues. (McNeese State University, Lake Charles, LA)

- The group concurred that post-tenure review process must be robust in order to confront an unproductive tenured faculty member; faculty colleagues may be more effective in delivering a message to this person than the dean, such as "I resent what you're not doing while I'm working hard"; Dean may need to say "Everybody thinks you're underperforming. Do you enjoy that status? How can we get you back on track? We're going to come up with a plan."

PRIORITIZING—How can we focus on the institutional mission?

- Recognize and curtail "mission creep" that stretches resources. Engage in strategic planning. Do an environmental scan. Examine the mission. Assess resources. Where are the mismatches? Jettison courses that are under-enrolled regardless of how long-standing or dearly held they are.
- Agree with other schools of nursing that each will teach within their areas of strength, perhaps eliminating duplication of programs.
- Convince college/university executive leaders that nursing is important to the school, i.e., that the nursing major contributes to liberal arts because students need those prerequisites. Talk to everyone on campus. Attend all possible meetings. Be visible and articulate. As a result of these types of activities, Villa Julie College in Baltimore is a leader in maintaining the college president's vision and strategic plan.
- Saint Xavier University in Chicago found federal funding to utilize local schools, students, and families for community-based programs. They also have a campus center to care for the elderly and increased emphasis on minority programs. Because service is a school priority, these activities offer student learning experiences while serving the community.
- Position your school well in the state. Faculty (not just the dean) should talk to legislators and other supporters whenever opportunities arise. (University of New Mexico)

- Join forces with other schools to approach legislators with a unified message.
- Encourage dean-faculty collaboration when deciding how resources should be allocated. Share resources among several disciplines in a school, with each partner supporting the initiative financially, such as a resource lab. Additional positive outcomes include joint research opportunities, interdisciplinary case studies, and joint programming. (Towson University, Towson, MD)
- Unusual organizational locations for the nursing program are not always negative, although that might be the first impression. For example, the nursing program at the University of Tulsa is located in the college of business, a situation that has afforded nursing excellent resources.

IMPLEMENTING CHANGE

- Start with data: local, regional, and national, such as that offered by AACN. Use the data to identify trends, compare programs, and clarify problems. People listen to data much more readily than emotional appeals. We must talk the same language as the people we are trying to convince. (Howard University, Washington, DC)
- As possible, hire assistant professors in a group so they form a cadre. This group has impressive credentials and accomplishments and sees things differently because they are new. They can support each other, lunch together, and as a group, cause "critical mass" for change and innovation. Ask them what needs to change and use them and their suggestions. (University of Wisconsin–Madison)

ISSUES AND CHALLENGES

- Realize that clinical teaching is labor-intensive (particularly for undergraduate students) and seek partnerships with clinical agencies.
- These partnerships can offer a faculty-sparing effect, but some faculty may need to resolve the issue of perceived loss of control.

- Counter the "we're too busy to precept students" argument by identifying and marketing specifically what the school can do for the hospital. For example:
- A student's good precepted experience in the hospital is a powerful recruiting mechanism for the hospital.
- Use of a problem-based service learning format solves actual practice problems at a clinical facility, directly helping the agency. (St. Joseph's College of Maine)
- Recognize that a clinical practicum precepted by a non-faculty agency staff member is not a hands-off endeavor. It remains labor-intensive for faculty, but in a different way. When utilizing clinical preceptors, several issues must be resolved in advance, such as how to jointly evaluate students and assign clinical grades. Suggestions: faculty and preceptor establish objectives together; faculty make clinical rounds and takes notes on students; preceptors identify problems and help faculty evaluate students; students keep logs which faculty member reads; faculty coordinate and validate preceptor availability for students.
- Utilize clinical simulation. Some systems are extremely expensive (e.g. $250,000 and a full-time operator) but are exceptionally realistic, down to mimicking "patient" gestures. (University of New Mexico)
- Patient simulation systems are particularly useful in physical assessment courses, such as graduate nurse practitioner courses. (California State University Long Beach)

UPCOMING TRENDS

- 66% of students in master's programs are preparing for the nurse practitioner role, and this will continue to be the primary pool of future faculty. They may be exceptional NPs but are not necessarily prepared to teach and will require faculty development in order to be fully successful. However, there are many ways to develop faculty: attend courses, earn a certificate, observe excellent teachers, read books, do educational research.
- Within the faculty, different members can and should be allowed to do different jobs, all of which contribute to the mission. This is contrary to our historical desire to have all faculty

doing the same type and amount of productive work, which may not be a useful strategy for the future.

AACN Task Force on Future Faculty

Kathleen A. Dracup, DNSc, RN, FNP, FAAN, Chair; Dean, School of Nursing, University of California–San Francisco, San Francisco, California

Doris S. Greiner, PhD, RN, CS; Associate Professor and Associate Dean for Academic Programs, School of Nursing, University of Virginia, Charlottesville, Virginia

Sheila A. Haas, PhD, RN, FAAN; Dean, Marcella Niehoff School of Nursing, Loyola University Chicago, Chicago, Illinois

Pamela Kidd, PhD, APRN, FAAN; Associate Dean of Graduate Programs and Research, College of Nursing, Arizona State University, Tempe, Arizona

Rose Liegler, PhD, RN; Dean, School of Nursing, Azusa Pacific University, Azusa, California

Richard MacIntyre, PhD, RN; Chair, Division of Nursing and Health Professions, Mercy College, Dobbs Ferry, New York

M. Dee Williams, PhD, RN; Executive Associate Dean and Associate Dean for Clinical Affairs, School of Nursing, University of Florida, Gainesville, Florida

Linda Berlin, DrPH, RN; Staff Liaison, Director of Research and Data Services, American Association of Colleges of Nursing, Washington, DC

Barbara K. Penn, PhD, RN; Staff Liaison; Director, Member Education; American Association of Colleges of Nursing, Washington, DC

REFERENCES

American Association of Colleges of Nursing. (1993, 1994). Faculty resignations and retirements (unpublished data). Washington, DC: American Association of Colleges of Nursing.

American Association of Colleges of Nursing. (1993–2002). Faculty age database (unpublished data). Washington, DC: American Association of Colleges of Nursing.

American Association of Colleges of Nursing. (1996). The essentials of master's education for advanced practice nursing. Washington, DC: American Association of Colleges of Nursing, p.3.

American Association of Colleges of Nursing. (1999a). Faculty shortages intensify nation's nursing deficit (issue bulletin). Washington, DC: American Association of Colleges of Nursing. Available from: http://www.aacn.nche.edu/Publications/issues/IB499WB.htm

American Association of Colleges of Nursing. (1999b). White paper: Distance technology in nursing education. Washington, D.C: American Association of Colleges of Nursing. Available from: http://www.aacn.nche.edu/Publications/positions/whitepaper.htm

American Association of Colleges of Nursing. (1999c). Defining scholarship for the discipline of nursing (position statement). Washington, D.C: American Association of Colleges of Nursing. Available from: http://www.aacn.nche.edu/Publications/positions/scholar.htm

American Association of Colleges of Nursing. (2000). Special survey on vacant faculty positions (unpublished data). Washington, DC: American Association of Colleges of Nursing.

American Association of Colleges of Nursing. (2002a). Accelerated programs: The fast-track to careers in nursing (issue bulletin). Washington, D.C: American Association of Colleges of Nursing. Available from: http://www.aacn.nche.edu/Publications/issues/Aug02.htm

American Association of Colleges of Nursing. (2002b). Faculty resignations and retirements (unpublished data). Washington, DC: American Association of Colleges of Nursing.

American Association of Colleges of Nursing. (2002c). Survey regarding education-practice partnerships (unpublished data). Washington, DC: American Association of Colleges of Nursing.

American Association of Colleges of Nursing. (2002d). Baccalaureate Education Conference (program session). November 14–16, Lake Buena Vista, Florida.

American Association of Colleges of Nursing. (2003a). Master's Education Conference, February 27-March 1 (abstract presentation). Amelia Island, Florida.

American Association of Colleges of Nursing. (2003b). Spring Annual Meeting, March 22–25 (program session). Washington, D.C.

American Association of Colleges of Nursing. (2003c). Hot Issues Conference, April 24–26 (program session). San Antonio, Texas.

American Association of Colleges of Pharmacy. (2003). Academic career seminar draws more interest. AACP News, 34 (2), 1–2. Alexandria, VA: American Association of Colleges of Pharmacy.

Anderson, C. A. (1998). Academic nursing: a desirable career? Nursing Outlook, 46(1), 5–6.

Anderson, C. A. (2002). A reservoir of talent waiting to be tapped. Nursing Outlook, 50 (1), 1–2.

Association of Governing Boards. (2002). Workload at Ithaca College: a faculty development model. AGB Priorities, 18, 4–5.

Berberet, J. & McMillin, L. (2002). The American professoriate in transition. AGB Priorities. Spring (18), 1–15. Washington, DC: Association of Governing Boards of Universities and Colleges.

Berlin, L. E., Bednash, G. D., & Alsheimer, O. (1993). 1992–1993 enrollment and graduations in baccalaureate and graduate programs in nursing. Washington, DC: American Association of Colleges of Nursing.

Berlin, L. E., Bednash, G. D., & Haux, S. (1991). 1990–1991 enrollment and graduations in baccalaureate and graduate programs in nursing. Washington, DC: American Association of Colleges of Nursing.

Berlin, L.E. & Bednash, G.D. (1995). 1994–1995 enrollment and graduations in baccalaureate and graduate programs in nursing. Washington, DC: American Association of Colleges of Nursing.

Berlin, L.E. & Bednash, G.D. (2000). 1999–2000 enrollment and graduations in baccalaureate and graduate programs in nursing. Washington, DC: American Association of Colleges of Nursing.

Berlin, L.E., Bednash, G.D., & Stennett, J. (2001). 2000–2001 enrollment and graduations in baccalaureate and graduate programs in nursing. Washington, DC: American Association of Colleges of Nursing.

Berlin, L.E. & Sechrist, K.R. (2002a). The shortage of doctorally prepared nursing faculty: a dire situation. Nursing Outlook, 50 (2), 50–56.

Berlin, L.E. & Sechrist, K.R. (2002b). Regression analysis of full-time master's prepared faculty in baccalaureate and graduate nursing programs (unpublished data).

Berlin, L.E. & Sechrist, K.R. (2003a). Percent of full-time doctorally prepared faculty over and under the age of 50 for 2002 (unpublished data).

Berlin, L.E. & Sechrist, K.R. (2003b). Percent of full-time master's prepared faculty over and under the age of 50 (unpublished data).

Berlin, L.E. & Sechrist, K.R. (2003c). Percent of full-time doctorally prepared faculty by age category, 2002 (unpublished data).

Berlin, L.E. & Sechrist, K.R. (2003d). Percent of full-time master's prepared faculty by age category, 2002 (unpublished data).

Berlin, L.E. & Sechrist, K.R. (2003e). Analysis of selected variables pertaining to full-time nurse faculty from the 1999 study of postsecondary faculty (unpublished data).

Berlin, L.E., Stennett, J., & Bednash, G.D. (2002a). 2001–2002 salaries of instructional and administrative nursing faculty in baccalaureate and graduate programs in nursing. Washington, DC: American Association of Colleges of Nursing.

Berlin, L.E., Stennett, J., & Bednash, G.D. (2003a). 2002–2003 enrollment and graduations in baccalaureate and graduate programs in nursing. Washington, DC: American Association of Colleges of Nursing.

Berlin, L.E., Stennett, J., & Bednash, G.D. (2003b). 2002–2003 salaries of instructional and administrative nursing faculty in baccalaureate and graduate programs in nursing. Washington, DC: American Association of Colleges of Nursing.

Billings, D.M. (2003). What does it take to be a nurse educator? Journal of Nursing Education, 42 (3), 99–100.

Bland, C., Seaquist, E., Pacala, J., Center, B., & Finstad, D. (2002). One school's strategy to assess and improve the vitality of its faculty. Academic Medicine (77): 368–376.

Brendtro, M. & Hegge, M. (2000). Nursing faculty: one generation away from extinction? Journal of Professional Nursing, 16, 97–103.

Brown, B.S. (2001). The multigenerational workforce: mixing it up at the coffee station. Review, 7–13; 19. Glen Allen, VA: Virginia Hospital and Healthcare Association.

Carnegie Foundation for the Advancement of Teaching. (2003). Carnegie Academy for the Scholarship of Teaching and Learning (CASTL) Higher Education Program. Menlo Park, CA: Available from: http://www.carnegiefoundation.org/CASTL/highered/index.htm

California Strategic Planning Committee for Nursing. (2001). Anticipated need for faculty in California schools of nursing for school years 2001–2002 and 2002–2003 (press release). Irvine, CA: Available from: http://www.ucihs.uci.edu/cspcn

Council on College Education for Nursing. (2002). SREB study indicates serious shortage of nursing faculty. Atlanta, GA: Southern Regional Education Board. Available from: http://www.sreb.org/programs/nursing/publications/pubindex.asp

DeYoung, S. & Bliss, J. (1995). Nursing faculty-an endangered species? Journal of Professional Nursing, 11 (2), 84–88.

Diekelman, N. (2002). Engendering community: Learning and sharing expertise in skills and practices of teaching. Journal of Nursing Education (41): 241–242.

Division of Nursing, Bureau of Health Professions, HRSA. (2001). The registered nurse population: national sample survey of registered nurses (unpublished special reports generated for the American Association of Colleges of Nursing).

Dorfman, L. (1989) British and American academics in retirement. Educational Gerontology, 15, 25–40.

Education Scholar Program. (2003). Available from: http://www.educationscholar.org/eds_about.htm

Fogg, P. (2003). The Chronicle of Higher Education, 59 (22): A8–A9.

Fong, C. M. (1993). A longitudinal study of the relationships between overload, social support, and burnout among nursing educators. Journal of Nursing Education, 32 (1), 24–9.

Furino, A., Gott, S., & Miller, D. R. (Editors) (2000). Health and nurses in Texas: the future of nursing: data for action. A report of the Texas nurse workforce data system. 3: (1), p. 5.21. Austin, TX: Texas Nurses Foundation.

Health Resources & Services Administration. (2001). Division of Nursing Nursing Workforce Diversity Program Directors Meeting, March 20–21, Washington, D.C.

Hecker, D. E. (2001). Occupational employment projections to 2010. Monthly Labor Review, 124 (11), 57–84. Available from: http://stats.bls.gov/opub/mlr/2001/11/art4abs.htm.

Hinshaw, A. S. (2001). A continuing challenge: the shortage of educationally prepared nursing faculty. Online Journal of Issues in Nursing, 6(1) Manuscript 3. Available from: URL: http://www.nursingworld.org/ojin/topic14/tpc14_3.htm.

Johnson & Johnson. (2002) Campaign for Nursing's Future. Available from: http://www.discovernursing.com

Kelly, N.R. & Swisher, L. (1998). The transitional process of retirement for nurses. Journal of Professional Nursing, 14 (1), 53–61.

Ketefian, S. (1991). Doctoral preparation for faculty roles: expectations and realities. Journal of Professional Nursing, 7(2), 105–111.

Levine, A. & Cureton, J. (1998). When hope and fear collide: A portrait of today's college student. San Francisco: Jossey-Bass Publishers.

Longin, T. C. (2002). Towards a 21st century academe. AGB Priorities. Spring (18),16. Washington, DC: Association of Governing Boards of Universities and Colleges.

National League for Nursing (1988). Nursing Data Review, 1987. New York: National League for Nursing.

National Opinion Research Center. (2001). Survey of earned doctorates. (Unpublished special reports generated for the American Association of Colleges of Nursing). Chicago, IL: National Opinion Research Center.

Nurses for a Healthier Tomorrow. (2000). Available from: http://www.nursesource.org

Oermann, M. H. (1998). Work-related stress of clinical nursing faculty. Journal of Nursing Education, 37 (7), 302–4.

Preparing Future Faculty Program. (2003) Washington, DC: Preparing Future Faculty National Office. Available from: http://www.preparing-faculty.org

Peterson's Colleges of Nursing Database. (2002). (Special database created for AACN internal research purposes). Lawrenceville, NJ: Peterson's, a part of The Thomson Corporation.

Pololi, L., Knight, S., Dennis, K., & Frankel, R. (2002). Helping medical school faculty realize their dreams: An innovative, collaborative mentoring program. Academic Medicine (77): 377–384.

Potempa, K. (2001). Where winds the road of distance education in nursing? Journal of Nursing Education, 40 (7), 291–292.

Porter-O'Grady, T. (2001). Profound change: 21st century nursing. Nursing Outlook (49): 182–186.

Rudy, E.B. (2001). Supportive work environments for nursing faculty. AACN Clinical Issues, 12 (3), 401–410.

Salary.Com. (March 2002). Available from: http.//www.salary.com

Spratley, E., Johnson, A., Sochalski, J., Fritz, M, & Spencer, W. (2001). The registered nurse population, March 2000. Findings from the national sample survey of registered nurses. US Department of Health and Human Services, Health Resources and Service Administration, Bureau of Health Professions, Division of Nursing.

Staiger, D.O., Auerbach, D.I., & Buerhaus, P.I. (2000) Expanding career opportunities for women and the declining interest in nursing as a career. Nursing Economics 18, 226–236.

Tanner, C.A. (2001). Competency-based education: The new panacea? Journal of Nursing Education, 40 (9), 387–8.

Tumolo, J. & Collins, A. (2001). Results of the 2002 national salary survey of nurse practitioners. ADVANCE for Nurse Practitioners. King of Prussia, PA: ADVANCE for Nurse Practitioners. Available from: http://www.advancefornp.com/npsalsurv01.html

Western Interstate Commission for Higher Education. (1998). Knocking at the college door: projections of high school graduates by state and race/ethnicity, 1996–2012. Boulder, CO: Western Interstate Commission for Higher Education.

University of California and the SAT (October 2001). Predictive validity and differential impact of the SAT I and SAT II at the University of California. Available from: www.ucop.edu/sas/research/researchand-planning

US Department of Education. National Center for Education Statistics. (2001). National study of postsecondary faculty (NSOPF: 99) public use data analysis system (DAS). Washington, DC: NCES 2001–203.

US Department of Education. National Center for Education Statistics. (2002). The condition of education: 2002. Washington, DC: US Government Printing Office, NCES 2002-025.

Vickers, J. (Winter 2002). Nurse staffing and patient outcomes: a reevaluation. Carolina Nursing, 6. Chapel Hill, NC: Carolina Nursing Research Chronicle.

White, K.R., Wax, W.A., & Berrey, A.L. (2000). Accelerated second degree advanced practice nurses: How do they fare in the job market? Nursing Outlook, 48 (5), 218–222.

Young, J. R. (2002). Homework? What homework? The Chronicle of Higher Education, 59 (15): A35–A37.

Zemke, R. (2001). Here come the millennials. Training, 38 (7), 44–49.

AACN White Paper "Faculty Shortages in Baccalaureate and Graduate Nursing Programs: Scope of the Problem and Strategies for Expanding the Supply" available from http://www.aacn.nche.edu/Publications/WhitePapers/FacultyShortages.htm

Index

Note: Page numbers followed by "f" and "t" indicate figures and tables, respectively.